Capucine ROUMIGUIE

Influence of dental occlusion on postural stature:

Capucine ROUMIGUIE

Influence of dental occlusion on postural stature:

Evaluation of diagnostic means from clinical cases

ScienciaScripts

Imprint
Any brand names and product names mentioned in this book are subject to trademark, brand or patent protection and are trademarks or registered trademarks of their respective holders. The use of brand names, product names, common names, trade names, product descriptions etc. even without a particular marking in this work is in no way to be construed to mean that such names may be regarded as unrestricted in respect of trademark and brand protection legislation and could thus be used by anyone.

Cover image: www.ingimage.com

This book is a translation from the original published under ISBN 978-620-2-54629-4.

Publisher:
Sciencia Scripts
is a trademark of
International Book Market Service Ltd., member of OmniScriptum Publishing Group
17 Meldrum Street, Beau Bassin 71504, Mauritius
Printed at: see last page
ISBN: 978-620-3-40287-2

Influence of dental occlusion on postural stature: evaluation of diagnostic means from clinical cases

Thank you,

        To my parents

These few words cannot tell you how much I love you. I would never have got to where I am today without you. From the first day I started school until now you have always been behind me, supporting me, helping me, supporting me and above all believing in me. You have always put your happiness after ours, you have given us everything and taught us everything, I couldn't have had better parents. I hope today to make you proud.

Mum, you're wonderful, a real example for me, so courageous, devoted, loving, intelligent (we don't congratulate you enough on your professional retraining, you've managed to return to school brilliantly) You've always believed in me, for you I've always been the best. Thank you for all your love, my success is yours.

Dad, the best without a doubt, you have always been my pillar in my school career, helping me throughout these years, know that this success is also yours because I could not have succeeded without you.

        To my brother,

Paul, my Paulus, my beloved little brother, I am very proud of you, you have chosen your path and I send you all my encouragement: go ahead, have confidence in yourself! You have all the capacities to become the best! Know that I will always be there for you. I love you very much

        To my maternal grandparents,

Papi and mami, thank you for all the love you have always given me, thank you for keeping me so well all these summers, thank you for spoiling me so much ! I hope I make you proud today.

        To my paternal grandparents

Thank you for giving me the best dad.

        In **Fabien**

It is during these years of étuszq that we met, more precisely during a quiet stay in the mountains !!! Since then you have been supporting me, supporting me and supporting me every day. We have already shared so many memories, but I hope to come again, when I'm with you, life is much easier and for that I thank you. Your bokit who loves you.

        To the Rabineau family

Uncle jean-pierre, auntie mary :. Thank you for having always believed in me and for bringing me so much love. I know that you will think of me strongly on the day of my defence.

Clément, benjamin, my beloved cousins, I wish you both a lot of love and professional success. See you soon to celebrate together

To my cousin

Charlotte is a cousin, but above all a friend! We will have lived so many things together and especially during those dental years! Even if your move to Bordeaux means that we see each other less, I hope you know that you can always count on me.

To my friends

Marine, sailor, my beco d'amour, since we met our friendship has never ceased to evolve; benevolent, faithful friend, on whom we can always count, wingman ! I remember as if it was yesterday, periods of revision where we reassured ourselves as best we could by doing our stats, but also our P2 interior! Today you are one of my dearest friends; we have so many shared memories but I know that the best is yet to come. I can't wait for us to meet at the end of the world to cut short your departure to New Caledonia! I don't know what I would do without you!

Diane, my dianus, our friendship was born within these walls, we have lived so many things together: a beautiful trip to Thailand, many stays in Hossegor and Montjoi (thanks to your family for their kindness and welcome), a crit (half), thousands of meals (accompanied by wines of course) but also one night flats, wingman evenings and I forget some.... So many good moments are behind us but I hope the best is yet to come. I hope that we will meet again at the end of the world because a year without seeing you seems impossible to me.

Clémentine, my roommate, I am happy to have shared this year of living together with you, you are a golden roommate but above all a golden friend. In a short time we have shared so many memories ! Thank you for being my friend and for putting up with me for a year. I know that our best moments are yet to come!! I can't wait to see you in Martinique or elsewhere because your absence might be difficult for you too.

Anais, pompéro, we discovered each other in Thailand and in one month (but what a month!!!) you became indispensable to me. Your good mood, your lightness make you an extraordinary girl, you are full of projects and I wish you with all my heart to realize them but above all to be happy.

Tatiana, tat, my ex roommate, my Breton, my friend. You also knew how to live with me with brio and from this year spent together was born a wonderful friendship. I think your laugh is the thing I will remember most from my dental years, it was the rhythm of our days (I think I speak for everyone!).

Dorothée, my dory, my partner, thank you for having been my big sister all these years.

Mathilde, Ma mathou, you are like a sister to me, I know that whatever happens I can count on you.

Léa, **my lélé,** I will keep in memory all the good moments spent in this faculty but especially in the cafeteria during the dental aperitifs !!! I wish you a lot of personal happiness.

Camille and Jachon, our meeting was late but I'm glad to have you, our gossip evenings over a good drink are a delight! Can't wait for the next one!

Hélène, the rock'n'roll girlfriend ! Always up for partying, I hope to spend more and more good times with you !

Caroline, this year a big program is waiting for us, sewing, sport, parties ! I don't know if we'll be able to do everything but in any case good moments are waiting for us !

Pauline, I wish you a lot of happiness in Nice! Hoping that you will come back from time to time to feast with us ! !

In the category of friends, **Jean, Pierre, Patu, Boy, Micha ,Labbé , Vivi, Px, Julien** you are at the top, I am happy to have met you during our dental years ! I wish you a lot of happiness and success, hoping that our weekends and evenings spent together will last a long time!

And finally thank you to all my classmates and those I forget for all the good times we shared during these five years.

To Olivier and Valérie

Thank you to Dr Dupont Olivier for taking me under his wing and welcoming me into his practice. I also thank you for supporting me and passing on your knowledge, in one year at your side I have already learned a lot.

My val, thank you for being a real surrogate mother at the practice, your support on a daily basis means a lot to me.

To **Dr SCHAMBRI -MANGENOT Jeanne-Marie**, thank you for the warm welcome you gave me during the summer 2014 replacement, I have excellent memories of it.

To **Dr COMBADAZOU** Jean-Claude, thank you for proposing this subject and for giving me the chance to work on it with you. You are someone who is very involved in your work and an example to follow. I hope that I will have the opportunity to learn a little more about occlusodontics from you.

To all those present today, thank you very much for being part of this day.

To our President of the Jury

Dean POMAR Philippe

- Dean of the Faculty of Dental Surgery in Toulouse,

- University Professor, Hospital Practitioner of Dentistry,

- Laureate of the Institute of Stomatology and Maxillo-Facial Surgery of the Salpêtrière,

- Habilitation to Conduct Research (H.D.R.),

- Knight in the Order of Academic Palms

Thank you for doing us the great honour of accepting the presidency of this jury.

We thank you for all that you have brought to us during our studies, please find here the testimony of our gratitude and our deepest thanks.

I would like to thank you personally for the trust you have placed in me over the years.

To our jury

Mr. Doctor CHAMPION Jean

- University lecturer, Practice, Hospital of Dentistry,

- Vice-Dean of the Faculty of Dental Surgery of Toulouse,

- In charge of the Prostheses sub-section,

- Doctor of Dental Surgery,

- State Doctor in Odontology,

- DU Implantology of the Faculty of Dental Surgery of Marseille,

- Diploma in Clinical Implantology from the Brânemark Institute - Goteborg (Sweden),

- Vice-President of the National Council of Universities (section: 58),

- Laureate of the Paul Sabatier University.

Thank you for having so spontaneously accepted to sit on this jury.

We thank you for your generosity in sharing your skills and your cheerfulness throughout these years.

Please find here the expression of our gratitude

To our jury

Mr VERGNES Jean-Noël

- University Lecturer, Hospital Practitioner of Dentistry,

- Doctor of Epidemiology, -Doctor of Dental Surgery,

- Associate Professor, Oral Health and Society Division, McGill University -Montréal, Québec - Canada,

- Master's degree in Biological and Medical Sciences,

- Master2 Research - Clinical Epidemiology,

- University Diploma in Clinical Odontological Research,

- Laureate of the Paul Sabatier University

We are very grateful to you for agreeing to sit on our thesis jury.

Please find here the expression of our sincere consideration.

To our managing editor

Mr. Doctor DESTRUHAUTFlorent

- Lecturer at the Faculty of Dental Surgery in Toulouse,

- Former university hospital assistant in Dentistry,

- Doctor of Dental Surgery,

- Doctorate from the Ecole des Hautes Etudes en Sciences Sociales, specialising in "Social and Historical Anthropology" (Paris),

- CES of fixed prosthesis,

- CES of Maxillofacial Prosthesis,

- DU Prothèse Complète Clinique (Paris V),

-Lecturer at the Faculty of Dental Surgery in Toulouse,

-Attached Practitioner of the Toulouse Hospitals in Prosthetics and Occlusodontics,

- Laureate of the Paul Sabatier University

We thank you for accepting the direction of this work.

Thank you for your teaching, your kindness and your availability. Please find here the expression of my sincere thanks.

To our co-director

Dr. Combadazou Jean-Claude Combadazou

-Dental surgeon

-Doctor of Odontological Sciences

-Attaché of the hospitals of Toulouse

We thank you for accepting the direction of this work.

Please find here the testimony of all my admiration for the passion you have for occlusodontics on a daily basis.

Thank you for the pedagogy, support, availability and kindness you have shown throughout the development of this work.

Contents

In recent years, much work has been done on the link between occlusion and posture, with contradictory results as we will see in the literature review.

While clinically this relationship between occlusion and posture seems obvious, it is much more difficult to assess from measuring instruments, as we were able to see in a previous work (Mémoire d'ODF by MOUNET Louis) within the ODF service.

The question we asked ourselves initially concerned the reliability of the instrumentation in posturology. Indeed, diagnoses are made thanks to this instrumentation without it being known from a statistical point of view whether these results are reproducible and significant for the same patient.

During this work, we will propose the following path: a reminder on occlusion and posture, then a review of the literature concerning the influence of occlusion on posture; a study on the validity of complementary examinations carried out in posturology before studying this relationship on the basis of 30 clinical cases.

A. Definition :

1) **The different theories**

There are several schools :

a) Gnathologists :

Within this school, there are also several currents, but they all take as their reference position the Centric Relation (CR), an articular position linked to the condyle/glenoid cavity relationship.

(1)(2)(3) (4)(5)(6)

The National College of Occlusodontics proposes the following definition: "The centred relationship is the highest reference condylar situation, achieving a bilateral condylar-disco-temporal, simultaneous and transversely stabilised coaptation, suggested and obtained by non-forced control, reiterative in a given time and for a given body posture and recordable from a mandibular rotation movement without dental contact". ». In the sagittal plane, this is the arc of rotation 1-II described by Posselt.

For gnathologists this Centred Relation must be :

- reproducible, i.e. the clinical information must be found identically on the articulator that simulates the joint system.
- non-dental, i.e. independent of dental contacts ;
- physiologically acceptable ;
- technically recordable.
- Okeson would add that it is a musculoskeletally stable position(1).

Unlike IOM, which can only be registered on dentate subjects, this centred relationship allows for the treatment of the edentulous and orthodontic treatment.

In these different currents we have :

For these authors, this concept allows :

-stability of each dental organ (tripodism); the relationships between the arches simultaneously concern almost all cuspid teeth with pit cusp contacts.

-a wide distribution of simultaneous contacts (reduction of the load supported by each element);

-a unique, reproducible, stable mandibular position: which allows anchoring ;

-a stable, symmetrical swallowing position ;

-protection of the TMAs during muscle contraction;

-The propulsion is guided by the sliding of the eight mandibular anterior teeth on the six maxillary anterior teeth, creating immediate disocclusion of the cuspid groups: the guidance is therefore without posterior obstacles, without anterior limitations.

-the laterality is exclusively taken care of on each working side by the mandibular canine which slides on the palatal side of the maxillary canine: this canine function thus ensures the immediate de-occlusion of the other teeth.

This gives rise to the notion of "mutual protection or disocclusion of protection". Each tooth protects its posterior neighbour and its contralateral tooth.

Concerning the degree of tolerance of the IOM position, this current of thought has gone from the notion of a single fixed position, "point centric", to a slightly freer notion: "short centric".

Main protagonists:(6)

PKTHOMAS, MCCOLLUM, STUART LAURITZEN, CELENZA, D'AMICO GRANGER, PAYNE, STALLARD SOLNIT, WIRTH,O' GUICHET

Other concepts have been developed from the gnathological school. These authors believe that there is a debate between occlusion in centred relation and IOM :

-For some of them, this debate can take place in the sagittal plane: **long centric theory.**

- For others, this can be done in the sagittal plane and in the frontal plane: **long and wide centric theory.**

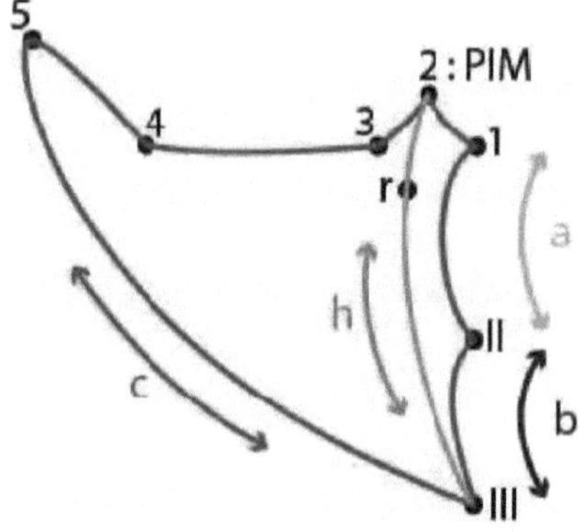

1. Occlusion of centred relationship
2. Maximum intercuspidation occlusion
3. Functional limit position
4. End-to-end incisal position
5. Mandibular propulsion
III. Maximum opening position
IV. Maximum rotation position

Figure 1 Posselt diagram(7)

These concepts of long and wide centric allow freedom of movement from point 1 to point 2 (Posselt's diagram) unlike gnatologists.

The notion of "group function" is also introduced, the balanced unilateral occlusion is obtained. During diduction movements, pressure is only distributed on the side towards which the mandible moves (working contacts), while the teeth on the opposite side are free of contact.

Main protagonists:(6)

PANKEY, MANN , SCHUYLER MORTON, MEYER, HANAU, RAMFJORD, DAWSON

b) Functional schools

These concepts reject joint RC as a reference position:

An American school was created under the impulse of Jankelson, the concept of "myo-centric" occlusion was born. It is no longer the joint that is taken as the joint reference but the manducator muscles.

In France, another functionalist school was born under the impetus of Jean Monod and Barelle, then Abjan a few years later. They called this muscular reference relationship the "usual functional relationship"(1).

Main protagonists:(6)

JANKELSON, SHORE, LE GALL JEAN MONO BARELLE, J.F LAURET

2) Conclusion: ideal occlusion?

In 2003, ANAES carried out a study on the review of the literature in order to clearly define the ideal occlusion, which led to the following conclusion: "no definition of the ideal occlusion can be established in a relevant manner".

There is therefore no a priori consensus on this definition. Webster defines dental occlusion as both :

- "The relation between the surfaces of the teeth when they are in contact" " i.e. the relation between the surfaces of the teeth when they are in contact.
- "the bringing of the opposing surfaces of the teeth of the two jaws into contact" i.e. the bringing of the opposing surfaces of the teeth of the two jaws into contact.

It emerges from these two definitions:

A static relationship: dental contacts

And a dynamic relationship, the mandibular movement that brings the mandibular teeth into contact with the maxillary teeth.

The definition of dental occlusion that we will propose is in perfect harmony with etymology and usage and is based on both Webster's definitions. That is to say, the shrinking operation on the one hand and on the other hand, the completion of the closure leading to the obstruction. This definition brings together dental movement and dental contact, but with the involvement of the neuro-muscular system, which is indispensable for the functioning of the manducatory system in the same way as the locomotor system.

Dental occlusion must therefore be taken into consideration :

1. The transition from the resting position to dental contact, the dynamic part of the occlusion corresponding to the approach of the dental arches thanks to the isotonic contraction of the masticatory muscles.
2. The dental contacts themselves which stop the upward movement of the mandible. This phase represents the completion of the closure, the so-called static stage of the occlusion. The contraction of the masticatory muscles then becomes isometric.

Whatever the movement studied, we must consider a reference position corresponding to the starting position of this movement and its return position. The usual position of the mandible is the so-called "resting" position, corresponding to this reference position from which the mandibular movements start and return(8).

In this so-called "resting" or mandibular posture there is a permanent minimum tonic activity of the masticatory muscles which is necessary as in all muscles of the postural tonic system and which opposes the action of the force of gravity exerted here on the mandible.

This position is therefore unstable; it will be subject to variations in relation to many factors such as the emotional factor, cold, abnormal dental contact, iatrogenic acts which will modify the activity of the muscles concerned(5) . As with the locomotor system, it will therefore have to be observed and recorded according to a given protocol.

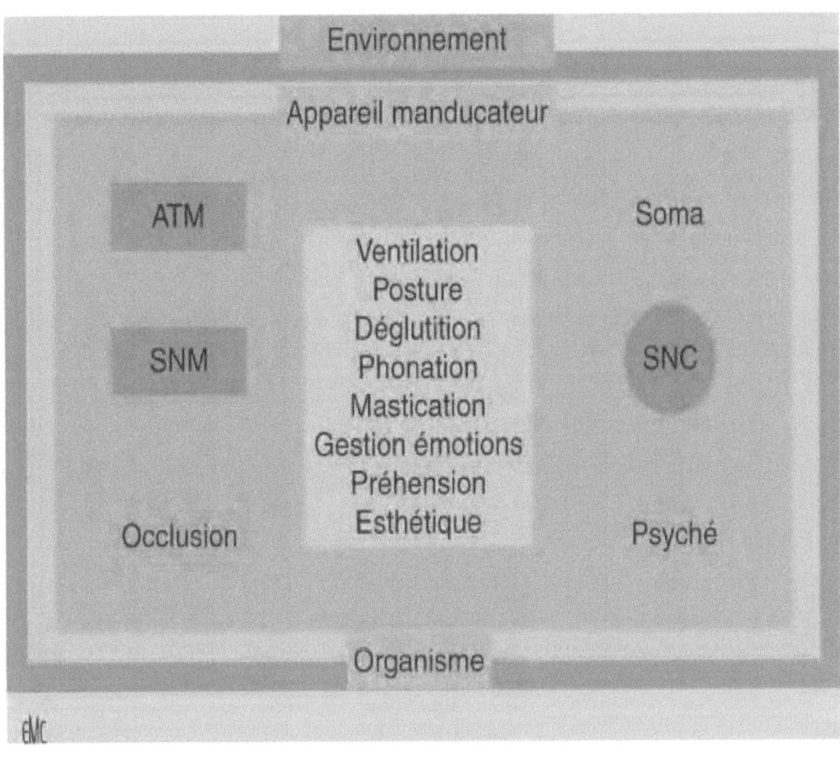

Figure 2 Slavicek's cybernetic system(5)

The recording of the intermaxillary relationship is more or less delicate depending on the chosen reference position. Indeed, when the practitioner chooses to record the IOM, it is a relatively simple act, the patient is brought to close in his usual occlusion position, it will then be necessary to check that the recording is correct.

The centred positioning is much more delicate...(9) This step requires correct handling by the operator to guide the patient without forcing the mandible.

There are different handling techniques, one of the most used is that of P.Dawson.

B. Role of occlusion

The functions of the occlusion most often mentioned in the literature concern its role in swallowing and chewing(10), and the fact that it allows the mandible to be centred, wedged or guided in the IOM (2)(5).

However, Gibbs and Lundeen (11) have shown that the forces exerted on the teeth during the final phase of chewing are the weakest in duration and intensity; the forces during swallowing are not much greater. The duration is only a few minutes per day. The question is therefore whether this intensity and duration alone is likely to cause any disease.

For Jean Claude COMBADAZOU, the physiological role of the occlusion is **to anchor the** mandible to the skull with the aim of :

- or to give a support point to the sus-hyoid muscles to raise the hyoid bone during swallowing.

- or to stabilise the cephalic end of the head at the front of the trunk by the only possible support point: the thorax.

Stabilisation is all the more effective when the anchorage is optimum so that the anterior, posterior and cross muscular chains are correctly linked together and integral in the action which is assigned to them.

1) <u>Anchorage</u>

This cranio-mandibular orthopaedic ratio normally corresponds to the maximum inter-arch contact point that the anatomical set of maxillary and mandibular teeth can offer. The number of contacts offered is highly variable depending on the occlusal concepts. Gnathologists recommend that each cusp in a pit should have 3 points of contact, known as tripodism. The number of contacts between 2 arches is therefore 172 points. The theories based on the concept of "centred freedom" propose 72 points of contact between the 2 arches (PANKEY-MANN-SCHUYLER concept). The reality seems quite different since a study by Valentin and Morin (12) shows that in young subjects with all their teeth on the arches, there would only be between 20 and 30 contacts.

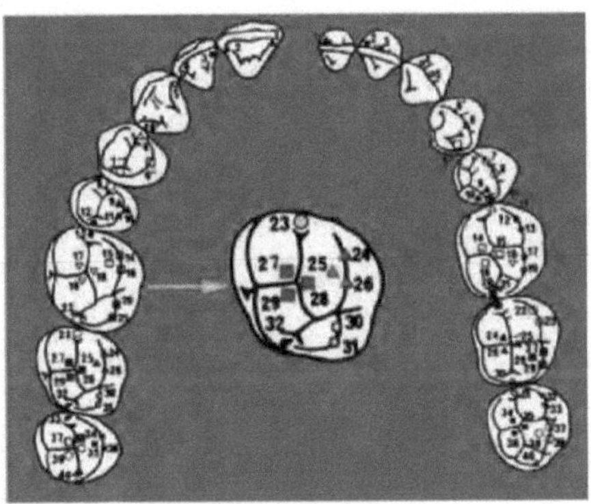

B. Dysocclusions

Dental dysocclusions or malocclusions are characterized by an abnormality of the occlusion of different origins:

- Genetics
- Congenital
- Environmental

They lead to structural alterations of the components of the manducational system and functional disorders. Since the role of the occlusion is to anchor the mandible to the skull, dysocclusions occur as soon as stabilisation is no longer effective in ensuring optimum anchorage, leading to asynchronous or insufficient contraction of the masticatory muscles.

Tables page 55 in "Practical occlusodontics"(2)

Anomaly	Consequences
Centering :	
-transversal	-Mandibular deviation
-sagittal	- Mandibular Retroposition (Angle Class II) - Mandibular propulsion (Angle class III)
-vertical	-Loss of DVO -Excess of DVO

For dunnage	Bite instability: dental migration
	Mandibular instability: - Occlusal interferences
	                            - Loss of posterior wedging
	                            - No previous shimming

II.   POSTURE

A. Definition

1) <u>Posture :</u>

If we look in the Larousse dictionary, posture is defined as "The position of the body or one of its parts in space. »

According to Webster, "posture is the development and active maintenance of the configuration of the different segments of the body in space, it expresses the way in which the organism confronts the stimuli of the outside world and prepares itself to react to them. It is the result of both tonic and phasic muscular activity. »

For Clauzade and Marty, it corresponds to a cranio-cervico-mandibular equilibrium which can be assimilated to a well referenced head in space.(13) The cranio-sacral-mandibular system, the primordial axis of our body, constitutes the fundamental referential of our verticality.(13)

According to Bernstein (1947) and his successors, they defined it as preparation for the movement(14)

From these definitions it is clear that posture is a static state that prepares for movement.

2) <u>Clinical concept of stability :</u>

Stability is a flexible concept, there are many ways for man to maintain himself near his equilibrium position(14).

If we look at the 2 diagrams below, the statokinesigram on the left has an area of 100 mm2, while the one on the left has an area of 50,000.

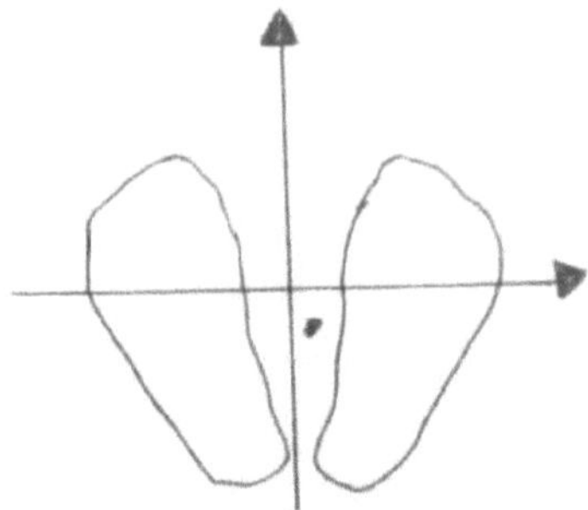

Figure 3: Statokinesiogram of a normal subject (14)

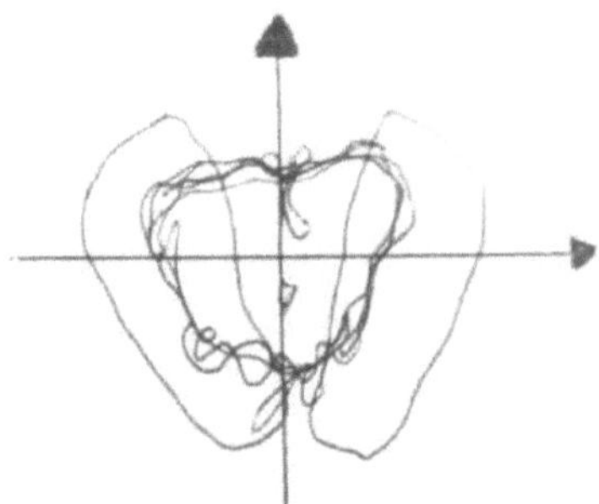

Figure 4: Balance according to Borelli's concept(14)

They both show a way of stability. The one on the left is that of the normal man who is almost motionless, the other that of a subject who explores his limits of stability on this sustentation polygon .(14) This flexibility of the concept of stability makes it possible to express and understand the nuances that exist between the different disturbances of balance, in particular thanks to its measurement.(14)

3) <u>Statics</u>

"Statics is the comfortable result of the container-content relationship, the aim of which is the more or less economic balance of the standing man"(15) The more economic this balance is, the more efficient it is.

3) **<u>Aplomb</u>**

"In physiology, it refers to the regular distribution of body weight on the limbs and the most favourable direction of the limbs considered as supports for the trunk and the execution of body movements"(3).

Or it is also "a state of equilibrium of the body resting on these limbs"(16).

4) **<u>Muscle tone</u>**

Tone is the state of muscle tone, or level of tension, of muscular "contraction".

The function of tonus is to ensure:(17)

- maintenance of antigravity and posture (through the play of tonic contractions),
- preparation for phasic contraction (tensioning of muscle elasticity).
- The basis of motor skills (voluntary or involuntary), language, non-verbal communication and expressiveness;
- support (and expression) of alertness, vigilance, motivation and intention (in relation to psycho-emotional and emotional factors).

In our study, we will focus on the postural tone which:(17)

- represents the minimum tonic activity for standing and maintaining static equilibrium, in different positions, as well as dynamic equilibrium.
- guarantees an optimum level of contraction for the action (state of "conductivity" of the voltage)
- is under reflex control but can also be controlled voluntarily.

5) **<u>Centre of pressure, centre of gravity and balance</u>**

The position of the centre of gravity (virtual, non-materialised point) depends on the distribution of masses and therefore on the body position; in the standing position. This centre is located just in front of the 3rd lumbar vertebrae. (15) As long as the centre of gravity remains aligned with the centre of pressure, stabilisation is effective. This stability corresponds to the average situation of a series of adjustments for which two tactics are possible: either the centre of gravity aligns with the centre of pressure or the centre of pressure aligns below the centre of gravity(14).

The construction of the human body, with a rather high centre of gravity, favours movement much more than stability (the ability to maintain stable equilibrium develops later than the ability to mobilise...). ,)(17)

The equilibrium corresponds to the projection of the centre of gravity in the "sustentation polygon" (17) . It is ensured by a set of pathways and nerve centres and manages the relationship between gravity, environmental stimuli and erect position(14) .

The man's position of equilibrium is the mechanical result of the torque produced by the forces of gravity / resistance. However, this balance is constantly compromised by stimuli from the environment but also from the organism(14) : unstable balance.

6) <u>Balancing</u>
(18)

"Balancing is the ability to maintain a posture in spite of adverse circumstances. It is therefore the result of the action of all the mechanisms which aim to maintain posture despite the causes which tend to disturb it when standing (static equilibrium) and when walking or gesturing (dynamic equilibrium). »

B. Role of posture

The role of posture is to :

- The "allow the movement of one segment while stabilising the other segments to ensure the station is maintained erected in the man's body"(18)
- (19) "Fighting gravity and maintaining an erected station";(19)
- "oppose external forces";(19)
- to "situate ourselves in the structured space-time that surrounds us";(19)
- to "balance, guide and strengthen the movement"(19).

C. Postural deficiency syndrome
(14)

The term 'postural deficiency syndrome' (PDS) was originally used by Martins Da Cunha, to refer to a set of tonic asymmetries and accompanying localised induced pain. (14) Gagey et al (1977) show that these tonic asymmetries are neither normal nor random. Therefore, on the basis of reproducible complementary examinations, it will be possible to correlate the results obtained with the symptomatology presented by the patient.

After the postural clinical examination, a test of asymmetrical thumbs, eyes open (97%), very often an unsystematised posturodynamic test (79%), associated in half of the cases with a blocked pelvic quadrilateral and, two times out of three, a homolateral Barré vertical, is found almost systematically. Nuchal gain is abnormal, above 45°. This is found in two thirds of the examinations.

D. The cranio-mandibular muscular system (2)(20)

The mandibular movements are performed by a muscular system comprising :

- The elevating muscles, powerful and with cranial insertion :
    o The temporal muscles and massage o The medial pterygoid

- Weak and hyoid insertion lowering muscles :
    o The supra-hyoid muscles (genio-hyoid, mylo-hyoid, stylo-hyoid and digastric muscles)
    o The infra-hyoid muscles (sterno-thyroid, thyro-hyoid, omo-hyoid): maintain the supra-hyoid muscles so that the mandible is lowered.

- A propelling muscle :
    o The lateral pterygoid: the upper head of the lateral pterygoid muscle has a double insertion, discal and condyle, to simultaneously control the position of the disc and condyle during closure of the mouth. This muscle, of which the disc would be a continuity, represents the disc tensor apparatus. This ensures that the joint is properly aligned during closure.

E. The muscle chains

1) According to BUSQUET
(15)(21)(22)(3)(23)(15)

Our musculoskeletal system does not actively move or hold itself, it is mobilised by the skeletal muscles and in particular by muscle chains. It is these which enable us to maintain balance and stability of posture and enable us to adapt to gravity.

BUSQUET defines these chains as "circuits in continuity of direction and plane, through which the organic forces of the body propagate".

Thus any work carried out at any point in the chain has repercussions on the chain as a whole. The movements are transmitted through each muscle within the chain.

The man can keep his vertical position, in relative immobility, thanks to the permanent adaptation of the tone of the different chains, saving the maximum amount of muscular work. These chains, with the exception of the posterior static chain, are chains of movement.

When it is necessary to compensate, the static adaptations will use the different chains, posterior straight, anterior straight, posterior crossed for a static purpose.

These muscular chains all relay to the scapular and pelvic belts which can deform, twist and tilt under asymmetrical stress in order to protect the spine.

The theoretical support for this concept of muscle chains is based on the notions of integration, sensory context and muscle starters initiating motor reactions under the dependence of low threshold mechanoreceptors (ROLL et al, 2000 and 2003). From this point of view, the chains are assimilated to sensory-motor loops, activated in a reflex manner from their ends using holding levers.

These chains are characterised by two operating principles, which are not contradictory, and whose purpose is movement.

They are going to be divided into straight muscle chains which are going to be divided into flexion and extension chains, subdivided into right and left, more structuring than the cross chains, which are rather intended for movement. These cross chains are divided into anterior and posterior right and left cross chains.

2) <u>According to STRUYF-DENYS</u>
(17)

«

- describes in a precise way and based on clinical observations, the different muscular and articular chains of the body;
- insists on the relationship between body tone and "shape" (attitudes), and proposes an associated study of craniometry;
- makes the link between chain "dominance" and psycho-behavioural impulses;
- develops a preventive as well as therapeutic educational approach based on these data

According to the principle of STRUYF -DENYS there are 5 muscular (and articular) chains (by way of influence...) distributed throughout the body and unifying, from head to hands and feet, all parts of the body, with important relays at the level of the pelvis.

These 5 channels are divided into :

- 3 fundamental, vertical chains (one of which is double), mainly concerning the trunk as a body axis, and referring to personal structure
- 2 complementary, horizontal (or "lateral") chains, mainly concerning the limbs and referring to the relational, dynamic axis, expression of the structure.

In the same person, the activity of these 5 channels is rarely completely harmonious and there is most often a "dominance" of one of them (in whole or in part), characterised by greater activity. The tone of this channel then becomes higher, with a tendency to shorten

and, in case of excess, to induce
The "deformations" in morphology, posture and movement, by progressive loss of
flexibility and freedom.
These dominances represent the specific mark of the expression, at the level of the body,
of the individual's psychic structure and behavioural tendencies. If they become excessive,
they then manifest the rigidity of these same characters".

There are other theories of chains, in particular that of BRODIE and LEJOYEUX.

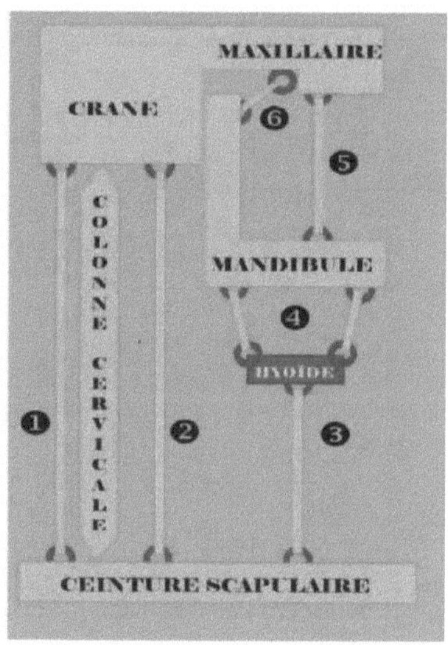

Figure 5: Brodie's diagram

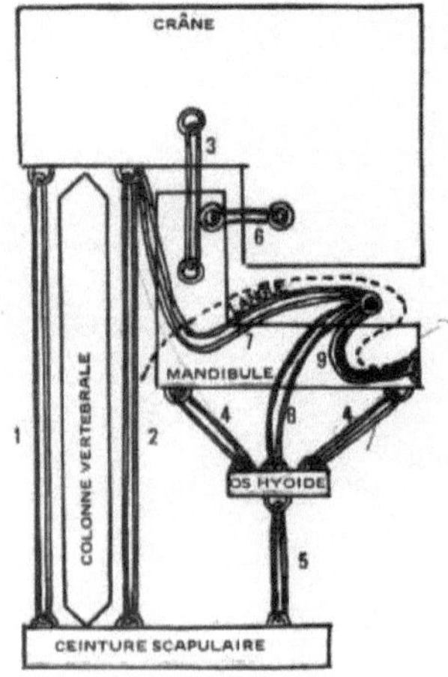

Figure 6: Lejoyeux's diagram

Literature review

The authors we have referenced are very divided on this relationship. Some believe that there is no relationship between posture and occlusion, while others believe that there is.

1) <u>No relation between occlusion and posture</u>

a) *" Dental occlusion and body posture : No detectable correlation"* (24)

This article published in "science direct" in 2006 will try to show through posturography if there is a change in posture when the dental occlusion is modified.

The study is carried out on 26 healthy patients, 13 men and 13 women aged between 21 and 38 years old.

The criteria for inclusion are as follows :

- good general health
- no vertigo due to central nervous system disease
- no symptoms caused by previous trauma or surgery
- the absence of any neurological abnormality, including vision assessment
- the absence of any particular episode of psychosocial and psychological stress in recent months
- the presence of a natural dentition and bilateral posterior wedging with canine and molar Angle I class +/- 2 mm
- the absence of a gap, an inverted bite and a significant overhang
- the absence of large restorations or cast restorations
- the absence of diagnosed temporomandibular disorders

Four different conditions were used during the passage on the posturology platform:

- Eyes open and mandibular resting position
- Open eyes and intercuspidation position
- Eyes closed and mandibular resting position
- Eyes closed and intercuspidation position

(The resting position means that the condyles are in a neutral and unconstrained position in the glenoid cavity and mandible at rest. The intercuspidation (unclamped) position is defined as the static closed position assumed by the mandible due to the meshing of the opposing teeth, independent of the centring of the condyle).

Each recording lasted 51 s, and four posturographic parameters were recorded:

- the mean absolute displacement of the centre of gravity of the theoretical point (ACOPD) (in mm)
- the projected balancing surface (area) (in mm2)
- the swing length (in mm)
- swing speed (in mm) VFY

(Only 90% of the projected points around the pressure centre (COP) were taken into account in the final estimation of the results).

A multivariate unidirectional covariance analysis (unidirectional MANCOVA) was performed to evaluate the differences between each parameter. The covariates were patient gender, age and weight. Sex and weight did not give any significant interaction, a new unidirectional MANCOVA analysis was then performed using age as the covariate.

Subsequently, four varied unidirectional united covariance analyses were carried out to separately assess the significant differences between the four posturographic parameters, i.e.: ACOPD, projected sway area, sway length, sway velocity

dRESULATES

- For the ACOPD parameter no significant results whatever the mandibular position or with eyes closed or open.
- For the other parameters the Bonferroni test found a $p < 0.05$ which allows us to accept the rejection of the null hypothesis and therefore to say that the results are significant.
- For these same parameters there is a significantly higher difference between closed eyes and open eyes.
- No significant difference, however, whether one is in the resting position or in the intercuspidation position.

Posturographic parameters among the diitcrcnt experimental conditions (n = 26>

Parameter	Condition	Mean ± S.D.
ACOPD (mm)		
	Eyes open RP	14.7 1 8.7
	Eyes open ICP	144 1 9.7
	Eyes closed RP	14.9 i 9.5
	Eyes closed ICP	111 1 11.2
	Diff.	NS
Sway area (mm2)		
	Eyes open RP	75.7 ±41.6
	Eyes open ICP	92.2 ± 64.0
	Eyes closed RP	137.3 ±94.8'
	Eyes closed ICP	138.8 ± 108.6*
	Diff.	;><0.05; S
Sway length (mm)		
	Eyes open RP	242.9 ± 65.7
	Eyes open ICP	255.4 ±79.1
	Eyes closed RP	330.9 ± 105.4*
	Eyes closed ICP	327.7 ± 103.8*
	Dill.	$p < 0.05$; S
Sway velocity (mm/s)		
	Eyes open RP	7J0± 19
	Eyes open ICP	7.4 1 2.4
	Eyes closed RP	9.5 1 3.1*
	Eyes closed ICP	9.4 1 3.0*
	Diff.	$p < 0.05$; S

Figure 7 results MANCOVA studies(24)

The ACOPD represents a static component, while the area, length and speed of swing represent dynamic components. The lack of significant results for the ACOPD suggests that this factor is not affected by dental occlusion or visual input suppression, at least in subjects without neurological disorders and in the age group considered in this survey.

Thus, this study does not show a detectable correlation at the posturographic level between dental occlusion and body posture, at least in the age range of the subjects included. Although this does not deny the existence of a correlation, more patients and more studies are needed.

b) Dental occlusion, body posture and temporomandibular disorders: where we are now and where we are heading for" (25)

This article was published in the "Journal of Oral Rehabilitation" in 2012, it aims to show, based on a review of the literature, the question of the relationships between dental occlusion, postural stature and temporomandibular disorders; but also the validity of the clinical and instrumental devices available (surface electromyography, kinesiography and platforms).

The biomechanical and neurological relations of the stomatognathic system with other regions of the body have been treated by an increasing number of researches in recent years (26)(27).

At present, the data in the literature has been based mainly on the effects of dental occlusion on the head and body (posture), while little information is available on the inverse effects of posture on dental occlusion.

Certain occlusal characteristics related to skeletal malocclusions (retrognathism, prognathism, hypo or hyperdivergence, facial asymmetry ...) are likely to lead to postural adaptation.
Particularly in skeletal Class II malocclusions, they are thought to be associated with cervical lordosis(28) However, no controlled investigation to date has included the effect of age as a possible confounding factor. This is important because age is the main factor influencing the degree of cervical lordosis, there is a direct proportional relationship, i.e. the lordosis increases with age(29).

The literature is also inconclusive about the influence of jaw position on the measured posture on postural platforms.
Available posturographic techniques and devices have failed to detect an association between body posture and dental occlusion (24)(30) or, when detected, it is often of little clinical relevance.
The most comprehensive evaluation published to date concludes that the usefulness of these instruments (surface electromyography, kinesiography, the stabilometry platform and posturology devices) on dental techniques is poor (31).

c)   <u>*1997 Milan Consensus Conference(32)*</u>

At this conference in 1997, it was reported that there was no scientific evidence to support a link between occlusion and posture. Thus, using occlusal treatment to prevent postural problems would not be justified.

2) <u>Proven relationship between occlusion and posture system</u>

a)   <u>*Article "clinical and instrumental treatment of patient with dysfunction of the*</u>
<u>*stomatognatic system: a case report" (32)*</u>

At another conference held in 2008, it was stated that the most recent scientific literature has provided little evidence to support the connection between posture, occlusion and neurophysiological integration of the body's mechanism(32) However, it is made clear in this article that occlusodontics today serves as a mainstay for diagnosis and therapy in dentistry, but that more detailed studies on occluso-cranio-mandibular relationships are needed to link this system to the rest of the body(4).

In this article, the T-Scan and a stabilometry platform will be used to treat a patient suffering from cranio-mandibular dysfunction(32) . This patient was suffering from both pain during mastication at the masseter level and cervical pain.

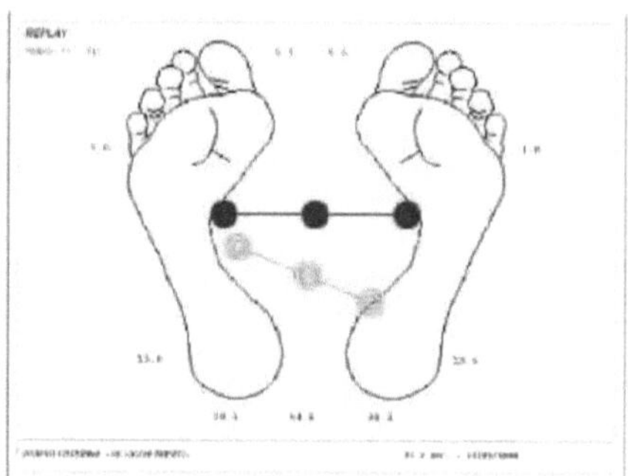

Figure 8 rearward projection of loads (32)

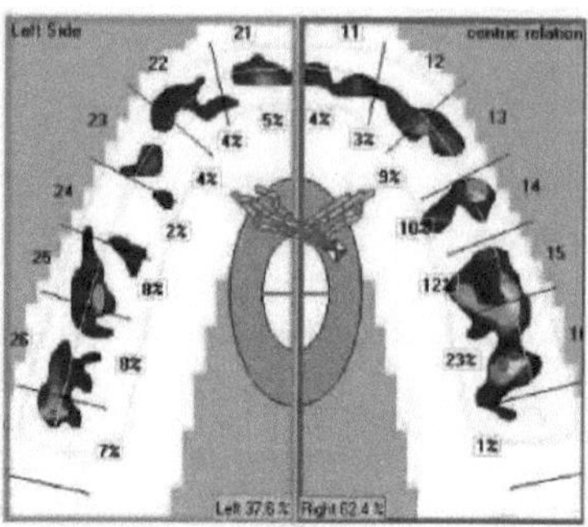

Figure 9 Dissymmetry of occlusal loads with 60%.

on the right sector and 40% on the left(32)

After treatment with occlusal trays :

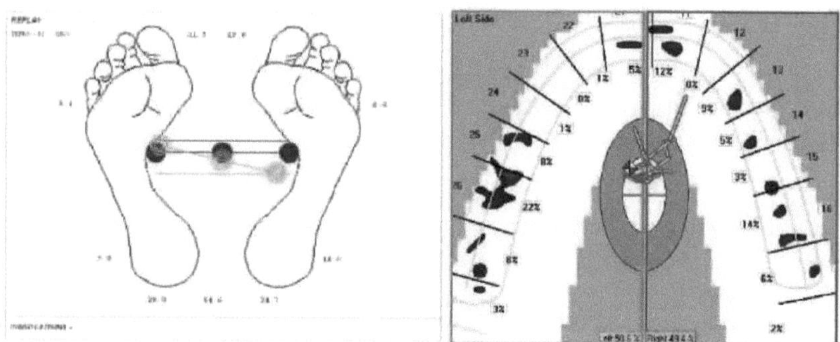

Figure 10 repositioning of the pressure centre (29) Figure 11 rebalancing of occlusal loads (32)

After a treatment carried out according to instrumental methods and protocols in accordance with the international literature, a significant reduction of pain in the masseters and a cessation of cervical pain is achieved after 4 months. Results verified at 6, 9 and 12 months(32)

There is a proven relationship between occlusion and posture, however, the single patient study is not very significant.

b)   <u>*"the spine journal" in 2014*</u>

This study investigated the effects of a temporary change in dental occlusion on the position of the spine, i.e. on posture. They compared this change in both statics and dynamics, i.e. walking(33) Previous research has shown that muscle activity and walking speed depend on the position of the cranio-mandibular system and vice versa(34).

This is a cross-sectional study which was carried out on 23 healthy patients, i.e. they all presented an absence of pain or dysfunction in the cranio-mandibular system.

To create a temporary bite modification, small 2 mm silicone panels were used on the left, right, front and both sides.

The experiment attempts to demonstrate whether or not a change in the symmetrical occlusion can significantly change the position of the spine (cervical, thoracic, or lumbar) when standing and walking.

To see these modifications, electrodes connected to a
250 kHz monitoring system (
desurface EMG

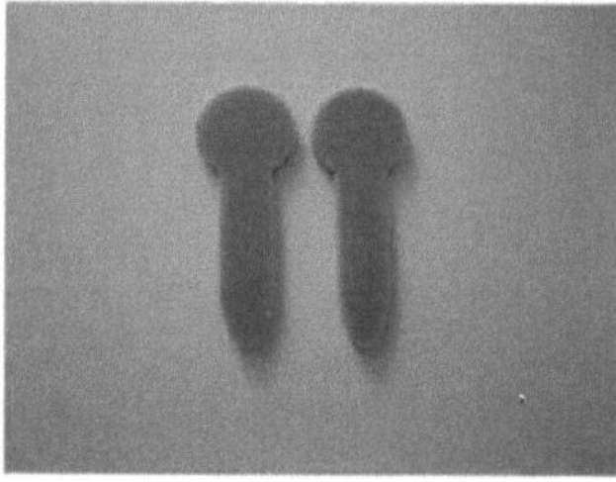

Figure 12 panneaux de silicone flexibles

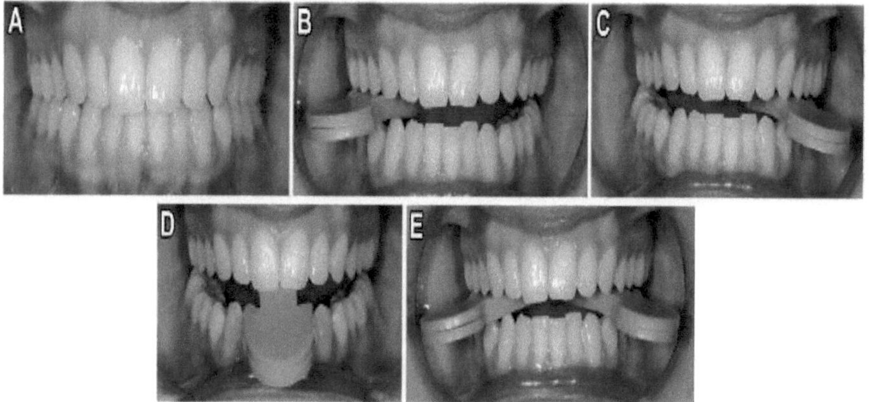

Fig. 3. (A) habitual dental occlusion; (B) right-side occlusional blocking of 4 mm; (C) left blocking; (D) frontal blocking; (E) symmetrical blocking.

) will be installed on the backs of the subjects, at cervical level,

thoracic and lumbar and these modifications will be observed in three planes: frontal,
sagittal and transverse.

/RESULTS :

*standing still :

For all subjects, in the usual position there is a left lateral flexion combined with a clockwise
torsion in the cervical sector, including a clockwise torsion in the lumbar and thoracic

regions. The occlusion block leads to a left lateral flexion in the cervical sector and a right lateral flexion in the other two sectors. In general, the thoracic region undergoes left-sided flexion due to occlusal interference but no torsion.

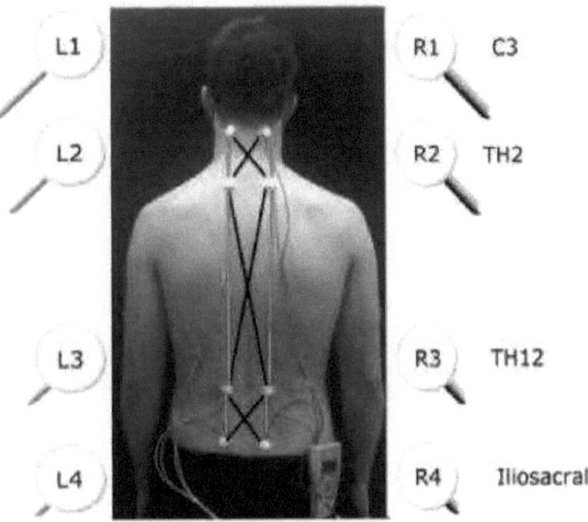

The comparison between the left and right sides of the body showed a significant difference in the cervical region.
In addition, there are more changes on the left side, once the silicone panels have been installed(33).

*Walking :

The usual upper body position undergoes a left lateral flexion and counterclockwise torsion in all three regions of the spine during walking. During walking tests with the silicone panels, changes in the position of the spine were detected.

The reduction of sensor distances in a sagittal, frontal and transverse plane during gait emphasises, a left lateral flexion in the cervical and thoracic sectors, and a constant torsion to the left, caused by manipulation of the occlusion. The change in left lateral flexion varies in the different regions of the spine during walking(33).

*Comparison of standing and walking :

During walking, there is significantly more cervical extension and a tendency to lateral flexion more to the left side in the cervical region than in the standing position. There is also a greater flexion in the thoracic and lumbar regions compared to the standing position. The changes in the lumbar region can be seen in all measurement conditions when walking. (6)

p Values of the comparison of measurement conditions between standing and walking for the left and right CS, TS, amt LS

| Standing/Walking | Habituai | | Right block | | Left block | | Symmetrical block | | Frontal block | |
	p (frontal, sagittal plane)	p (transverse plane)	p (frontal, sagittal plane)	p (transverse plane)	p (frontal, sagittal plane)	p (transverse plane)	p (frontal, sagittal plane)	p (transverse plane)	p (frontal, sagittal plane)	p (transverse plane)
CS left	.001	,001	,07	,01	.62	,19	.22	.03	,œ	,001
CS right	.001	.02	.08	.05	,13	.60	.12	.64	.04	.13
TS left	,99	.71	.01	.22	.56	,89	.05	.78	.43	.25
TS right	.19	.46	.15	.04	.85	,08	.05	.26	,02	.03
LS left	.01	.001	.001	JÜOI	.001	.001	.001	.001	,001	.001
LS right	.001	,001	.001	,001	YES	(MI	,001	.1101	.001	,001

We see here that out of 23 patients, the modification of the occlusion modifies the postural sature.

b) *In the book "new approach to cranio-mandibular dysfunction" by Pierre-Hubert DUPAS (35)*

In this book he highlights the relationship between posture and occlusion via the nervous network. In fact, various anatomical and physiological studies have highlighted the nervous connections between the trigeminal ganglion and the III, IV and VI pairs of cranial oculomotor nerves controlled by the oculomotor nucleus.

During dental contact, the branches of the cranial nerves V2 and V3 from the periodontal receptors transmit information to the trigeminal ganglion, which then sends stimuli jointly to the sensory nucleus of the V and to the oculomotor nerves. The periodontal information then reaches the sensory core of the V, then the reticular formation which controls the muscles of the scapular belt and those of the cervical and body posture.

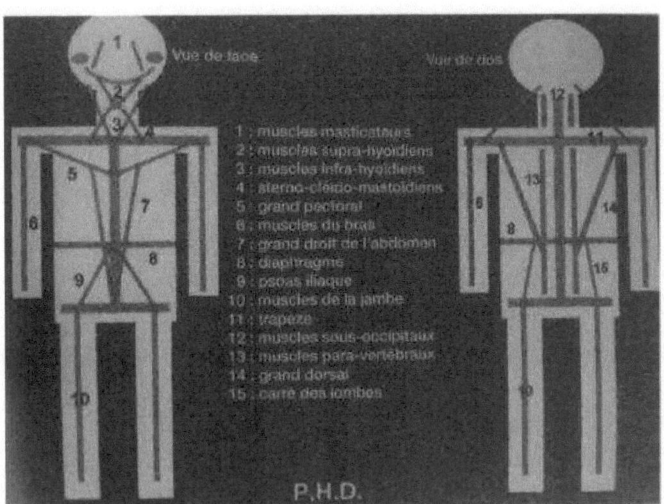

Figure 13 diagram of main muscle postures(35)

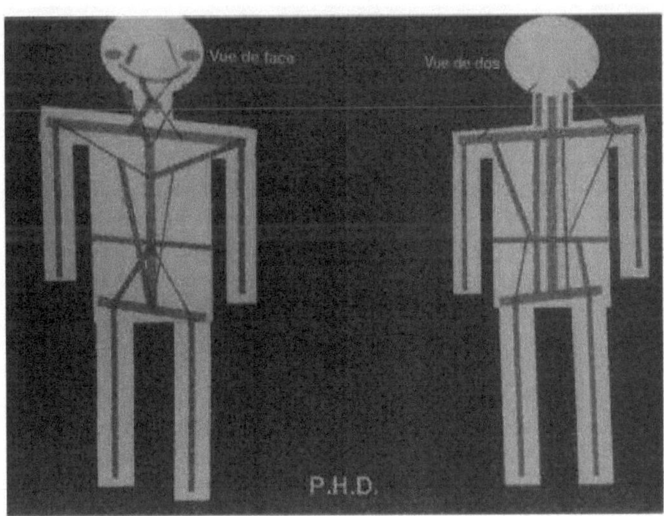

Figure 14 Homolateral belt tilting (35)

The schematic representations above represent the hyoid bone, the mandible, the scapular

and pelvic girdle which are entities here, the spine, the masticatory muscles and the main muscles of interest to the posture and the diaphragm. The diagram of the main muscles connecting the scapular and pelvic belts together explains why disorders of one reflect on the other. [See II.A]

c) *"Effects of different jaw relations on postural stability in human subjects "*[36]

This article was published in "neuroscience letters" in 2004. The authors studied the effects of different mandibular positions on postural stature in a sample of 95 subjects (23 men and 72 women aged 18 to 52 years).

All subjects were voluntary, asymptomatic, without information about the purpose of the study. A preliminary investigation was carried out in order to exclude signs and/or symptoms of temporomandibular disorders and psychiatric disorders.

Subjects underwent computerised postural and stabilometric analysis using a stabilometric platform. The recordings were made in three mandibular positions:

- intercuspidation position.
- resting position or mandibular position (this is the position occupied by the mandible when the head is straight, while the muscles concerned, particularly the lifts and depressors, are in a state of equilibrium and minimal tonicity, while the condyles are unstressed in their glenoid cavity), the unstressed position in the glenoid fossa)
- the myocentric position or myocentric occlusion (this is a position established along the neuromuscular trajectory, more commonly a position which is between 1 and 2 mm on the vertical closing path of the physiological resting position. This position occurs when the postural and masticatory muscles are simultaneously at their resting length and in a balanced tone relative to each other. Myocentric occlusion is obtained by transcutaneous electrical neural stimulation (TENS) technique, according to Jankelson (37)(38)(39)) determined respectively by the meshing of the teeth, the position of the joints, and the contraction of the muscles.

For each topic, three different recordings were made on the platform:

- the first in the position of maximum ntercuspidation.
- the second one with 8 mm cotton rolls which allow the resting position to be achieved.
- the third with orthoses that were made once the myocentric position was found

All subjects showed variations in body posture in different mandibular positions. Statistical analyses confirmed that the postural variations in the different mandibular positions were significant: in particular, the SKN multiple comparison test showed that the myocentric position improved the postural balance in the frontal plane compared to the other positions of the jaw.

d) _A rt i c le "Effect of Body Posture on Malocclusion "(40)_

This study was conducted to discover the association between body posture and the type, severity and location of the malocclusion. The sample includes 952 children (234 boys, 718 girls) between the ages of 12 and 15 years in the city of Karak in southern Jordan between September 2013-February 2014. The dental health component (DHC) based on the index of orthodontic tratment need (IOTN) was used to determine the type, severity and location of the malocclusion. They were treated separately, study models were taken of all the pupils and digital photos (frontal views) were taken.

The prevalence of asymmetry in the frontal plane is 38.8% (32.8% of boys, 40.7% of girls), which is close to the result found by Perillo 41.3% (male 44.2%, 38.4% of women).Perillo et al based their study on Angle's classification and the presence of crossbite, and other types, such as severity. However the location of the malocclusion was not considered. This may be insignificant in terms of the value of p, but in this study they relied on IOTN DHCs to determine the type and severity of the malocclusion and its location.

Grade 1 No treatment required. Extremely minor malocclusions, including displacements less than 1 mm	
Grade 2 Little need	
2.a	Increased overjet > 3.5 mm but $\leq$ 6 mm (with competent lips)
2.b	Reverse overjet greater than 0 mm but $\leq$ 1mm
2.c	Anterior or posterior crossbite with $\leq$ 1mm discrepancy between retruded contact position and intercuspal position
2.d	Displacement of teeth > 1mm but $\leq$ 2mm
2.e	Anterior or posterior open bite > 1mm but $\leq$ 2mm
2.f	Increased overbite $\geq$ 3.5mm (without gingival contact)
2.g	Prenormal or postnormal occlusions with no other anomalies. Includes up to half a unit discrepancy
Grade 3 Borderline need	
3.a	Increased overjet > 3.5 mm but $\leq$ 6 mm (incompetent lips)
3.b	Reverse overjet greater than 1 mm but $\leq$ 3.5mm
3.c	Anterior or posterior crossbites with >1mm but $\leq$ 2mm discrepancy between the retruded contact position and intercuspal position
3.d	Displacement of teeth >2mm but $\leq$ 4mm
3.e	Lateral or anterior open bite > 2mm but $\leq$ 4mm
3.f	Increased and incomplete overbite without gingival or palatal trauma

Grade 4 Treatment required

4. aIncreased   oveijet > 6mm but < 9 mm

4.   b Reverse overjet > 3.5 mm with no masticatory or speech difficulties

4.   c Anterior or posterior crossbites with > 2 mm discrepancy between the returned contact position and intercuspal position

4.   d Severe displacements of teeth > 4

4.   e Extreme lateral or anterior open bites > 4 mm

4.f Increased and complete overbite with gingival or palatal trauma

4.h Less extensive hypodontia requiring pre-restorative orthodontics or orthodontic space closure to obviate the need for a prosthesis

4.1   Posterior lingual crossbite with no functional occlusal contact in one or more buccal segments

4.m Reverse oveijet > 1 mm but < 3.5 mm with recorded masticatory and speech difficulties

4.t Partially erupted teeth, tipped and impacted against adjacent teeth

4.   xExisting supernumerary teeth

Grade 5 Treatment required

5. aIncreased   oveijet > 9 mm

5.   h Extensive hypodontia with restorative implications (more than one tooth missing in any quadrant, requiring pre-restorative orthodontics)

5.1   Impeded eruption of teeth (apart from 3rd molars) due to crowding, displacement, the presence of supernumerary teeth, retained deciduous teeth, and any pathological cause

5.   m Reverse oveijet > 3.5 mm with reported masticatory and speech difficulties

5.   p   Defects of cleft Up and palate

5.   sSubmerged deciduous teeth

Figure 15 Components of dental health according to IOTN(40)

Using IOTN's DHC, the following results can be found:

- The relationship between the frontal plane and the type of malocclusion is not statistically significant (p-value=0.17).
- For the relationship between the location of the malocclusion and the frontal plane the result is again not significant (p-value=0.14).
- **However, for the link between the severity of the malocclusion and the impact of the frontal posture, the results show a statistically significant value for the boy with a p=0.01.**

In this article, if we consider that about 33% of boys have frontal plane asymmetry, we consider this study to be significant for about 77 people.

This study could also be placed in the category <u>no link between occlusion and posture</u> as it is not significant for either type or location or for girls.

IV. VALIDATION OF THE INSTRUMENTATION FOR STABILITY MEASUREMENT

A. In occlusodontics

1) <u>The K7 Kinesiograph Myotronics Inc. system</u>

The K7 evaluation system has three technologies: for measuring, displaying and storing objective data on the physiological, anatomical and functional state of the cranio-musculo-mandibular system. (41)

With this system the patient will first undergo transcutaneous electrical neurostimulation to relax the muscles and relieve pain. At the same time during this stimulation, muscle activity is recorded by surface electromyography. Once the muscle activity is reduced to a sufficient degree, a recording of the mandibular movements is made.

This system will be described very quickly, and is only of interest here to explain how the treatment of patients was carried out.
Indeed this system will allow us to place the mandible in a neuromuscular equilibrium position, a position which will be fixed by mandibular gutters.

Figure 16(42)

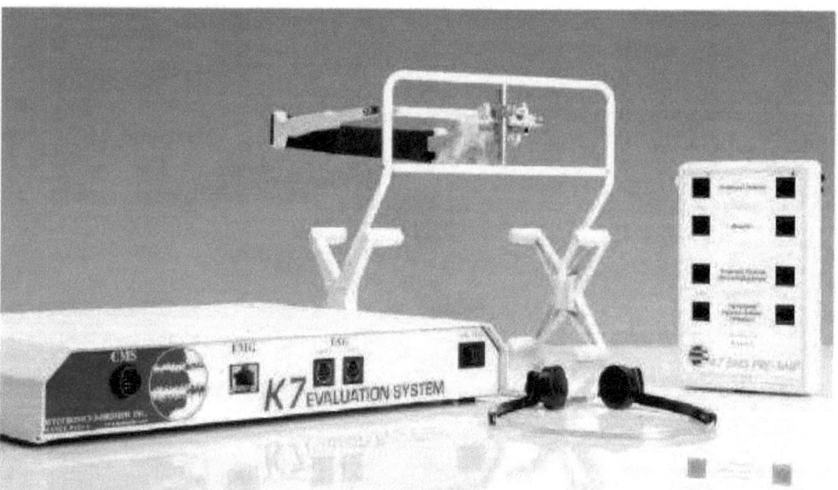

It is an evaluation system with patented technology that provides the data necessary to objectively measure occlusal function in three dimensions. (43)

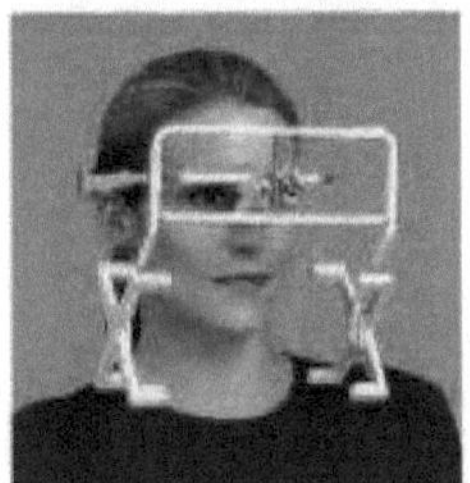
Figure 17(41)

It uses a magnet positioned at the lower BIC coupled with a sensor that is attached around the skull. This magnet-sensor couple system will allow the movement of the jaw to be followed by a computer program. It can determine when the muscle fibres are in their optimal position, i.e. when they are in balance and expend the least amount of energy to function.

Using high-quality bipolar surface electrodes, surface EMG data can be taken from eight muscle sites simultaneously and in real time. The programme allows the electromyographic data to be taken either at rest or in function. All eight sites can be displayed simultaneously, for a period of 15 seconds (the width of the visual screen). These analyses provide an objective measurement of the electrical activity of the manducatory muscles. (41)

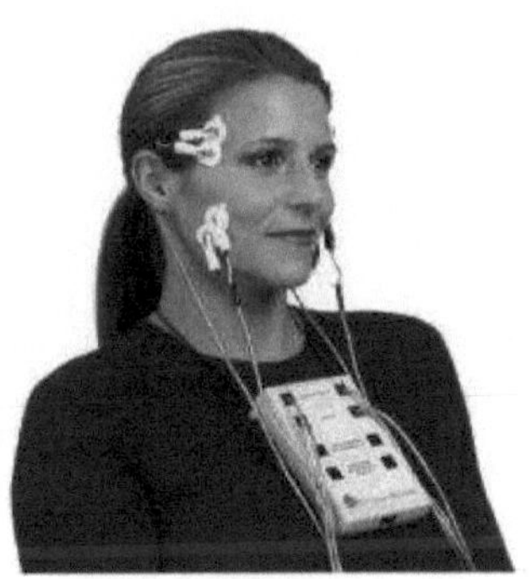
Figure 18 (44)

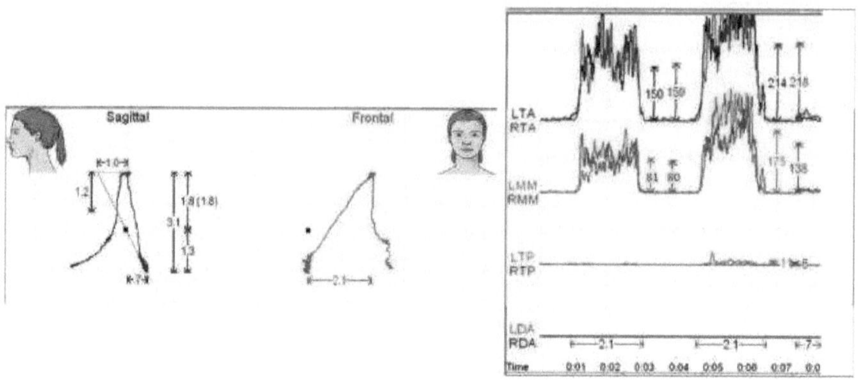

Figure 19 patient dr combadazou

B. In posturology

1) <u>Stabilometric or postural platform</u>

a) *Standard 85 and computerized standard platform (45)f14)*

In the 1970s, the international posturographic society founded a Standards Committee chaired by Kapteyn. The few clinicians who participated in the work of this society tried to make their problem clear: a doctor cannot make a stabilometric recording of his patients before they are ill! Whereas a fundamentalist can record his test subjects before and after the manipulations he imposes on them. Doctors therefore need statistical standards to place their patients in a distribution, fundamentalists do not.

The members of the French Posturology Association, have worked for a standardised clinical stabilometry platform (AFP, 1984). They immediately undertook the drafting of specifications for the construction of a standard platform.

Several guidelines guided their choices:

- The platform was intended for clinicians, not especially fundamentalists,

- its cost should allow for its wide dissemination,

-performance would be limited to the clinical study of what had already been studied in

46

the laboratory.

We will however give some characteristics of the platform :

- To measure the forces, it uses strain gauges because piezoelectric quartz crystals do not pass the continuous band; however, the frequencies studied in stabilometry go down to very low bands (0.04 Hz). The platform rests on three gauges: three points determine a plane and experience shows that it is very difficult to locate the tops of four gauges in the same plane.
- The surface of the platform is hard so that the contacts of the baroreceptors of the plantar sole are not blunt.
- Force measurements are only made 5 times per second. This very slow sampling rate (5Hz) may come as a surprise, but studies of various sampling rates have shown that for the moment and in clinical stabilometry it is useless to increase it.
- The recording time is 51.2 sec.

b) *Standardised records(14)*

The normal values of the stabilometric parameters have been studied and published (Standard 85) for two examination situations: successively eyes open and eyes closed. It is these two situations that are used to compare the patient's performance with that of the normal reference populations.

The subject's feet, bare, must be placed precisely on the platform, heels two centimetres apart, feet at 30° apart, and in such a way that the barycentre of its sagittal polygon is located on the sagittal axis of the platform at a known distance behind its electrical centre (this distance, generally four centimetres, depends on the software used).

The success of this standardised stabilometry is based on a semantic wager, i.e. each recording must be made in the same way. The patient will be asked to be immobile, relaxed, with his arms at his side, to look at a target in front of him, without staring at it, and to count slowly out loud until we say stop: all this information is given by Standard 85.

c) *Signal processing(14)*

The number of parameters that can be extracted is considerable, Gagey and Weber will limit themselves to two representations, the statokinesiogram and the stabilogram, six parameters :

- Xmoyen
- Ymoyen
- Surface
- LFS
- AN02
- VFY
- Romberg Quotient
- 6 functions

In the experimentation that will come later we will limit ourselves to Xmoy, surface, LFS, VFY and ampX/amp Y. Only the first four parameters are standardised, however we have kept ampX/ampY because this ratio also expresses the surface but in a more precise way (information given by the creator of the SATEL postural table).

Standard 85 defines normal values :

Xmoy	Eyes open	Eyes closed
Average	-1,1	-0,3
Lower limit	-9,6	-10,5
Upper limit	-11,7	-11,1

Surface	Eyes open	Eyes closed
Average	91	225
Lower limit	39	79
Upper limit	210	638

LFS parameter	Eyes open	Eyes closed
Average	1,00	1,00
Lower limit	0,72	0,70
Upper limit	1,39	1,44

VFY parameter	Eyes open	Eyes closed
Average	-0,00	-0,00
Upper limit	-2,61	-4,73
Lower limit	-3,59	-4,86

2) **Experimentation**

(a) Validity of the instrumentation and use of the Standards 85

If we rely on the values of STANDARDS 85, we can then compare the performance of patients to these standards and assess the quality of their postural system.

This would then allow us to use the device in the office to help diagnose the influence of occlusal disorders on posture and vice versa. Based on this postulate, Dr Combadazou wanted to check whether on healthy subjects (these three subjects are considered healthy since they are asymptomatic and have had neither occlusal nor postural treatment) the examinations for each of them were comparable over time and over one day, and whether the values recorded were comparable to those of standard 85.

With these two assistants, they registered several times a day for several weeks on a SATEL platform. About 40 recordings were made for each subject, with a change of observer. This number allows us to use the normal law and to find the confidence interval for each average when considering a risk index a= 0.05, i.e. out of 95%(46).

The formula used is as follows.

Thanks to the table of the Normal Law we will be able to find z: if we set our risk index at 0,05 we have 1-0,05/2= 0,975 and if we refer to the table we find z=1,96.Excel then calculates the results for each average.

Quantiles u(/3) of order fi of the law X(0,1), defined by $(u(0)) = fi- For fi < 0.5, use u(fi) - u(l fi)

	1.2816	1.6449	1.96	2.3263	2.5758	3.0902	3.2905	3.8906
r *(xF	0.9	0.95	0.975	0.99	0.995	t. 999	0.9995	0,99995

Patient 1:	number of registrations	standard deviation	average	risk of error	IC min. value	IC max. value
Xmoy	39	4,8339895	2,09049487	5%	0,573341555	3,607648188
Surface	39	1312,46572	806,674468	5%	394,7555506	1218,593385
VFY	39	2,8198397	3,471117949	5%	2,586169466	4,356189508
LfS	39	0,34954727	2,10642641	5%	1,996720587	2,216132233
ampX/ampY	39	0,2259889	1,04358974	5%	0,972662859	1,114516628

(Appendix 1)

Patient 2:	Xmoy	Surface	VFY	LfS	ampX/ampY
number of registrations	45	45	45	45	45
standard deviation	3,70502902	24,6185065	1,72083806	0,18223987	0,25790081
average	6,303172	132,468918	-3,73370644	1,41738156	1,18688889
risk of error	5%	5%	5%	5%	5%
IC min. value	5,220638291	125,2758941	-4,236500133	1,364134792	1,111535546
IC max. value	7,385705709	139,6619423	-3,230912756	1,470628319	1,262242232

(Annex 2)

51

Patient 3:	Xmoy	Surface	VFY	LfS	ampX/ampY
number of registrations	46	46	46	46	46
standard deviation	3,29616739	336,888692	1,73942003	0,13937032	0,44590721
average	2,2221963	225,310254	-9,97783543	1,19501761	1,57608696
risk of error	5%	5%	5%	5%	5%
IC min. value	1,279837265	128,995332	-10,47512759	1,155172279	1,448604145
IC max. value	3,164555344	321,6251754	-9,480543277	1,234862938	1,703569768

(Appendix 3)

Compared to the data of the STANDARD 85 :

value of the	Lower limit	Upper limit
Xmoy	-11,1	-10,5
S	79	638
LfS	0,7	1,44
VfY	-4,86	-4,73

Patient 1	Lower limit	Upper limit
Xmoy	-7,01	9,89
S	468,19	2372,81
LfS	0,9	1,4
VfY	-4,06	7,5

Patient 2	Lower limit	Upper limit
Xmoy	-1,35	12,53
S	87,63	188,06
LfS	0,57	0,9
VfY	-7,1	-0,06

Patient3	Lower limit	Upper limit
Xmoy	-6,06	8,57
S	108,98	790,23
LfS	0,45	0,83
VfY	-6,17	-14,06

To begin with, it can be noted that the extreme values of the surface are so far apart that one may wonder whether in our case, these values are precise enough to be used as an element of comparison.

The values of the 3 subjects are for some of them above the normal values:

-In the case of patient 1, only the LfS values are good.

-In the case of patient 2, the surface and LfS are good.

-In the case of patient 3, only the surface value is good.

Furthermore, if we look at the results we see that all the means fall within the confidence interval (CI) and therefore the results are significant, i.e. for the same patient the data are in agreement, but there is no correspondence between individuals. It can be deduced here that the results are significant intra-person but not inter-person.

It seems difficult from these data to say whether a patient is healthy or not, because the differences between people are too great (conf VI.D.1) in our case the values of standard 85 are not precise enough for us to be able to use them.

Ces résultats se vérifient sur les graphiques.

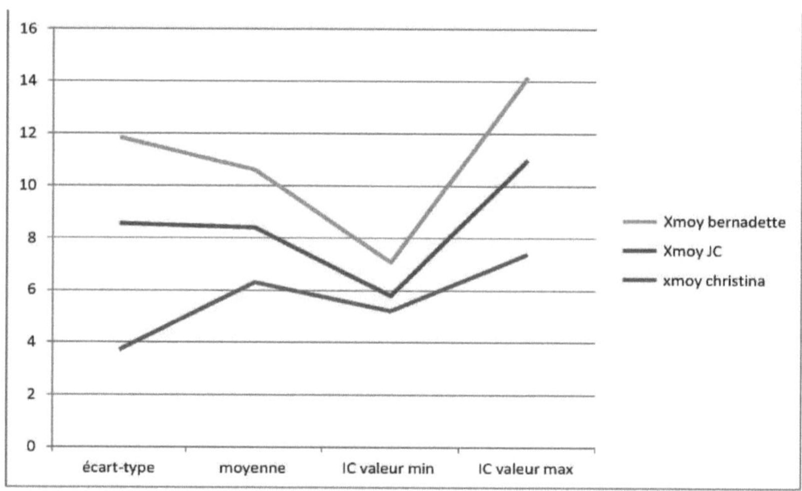

Figure 21: Comparison of the Xmean values between the 3 subjects

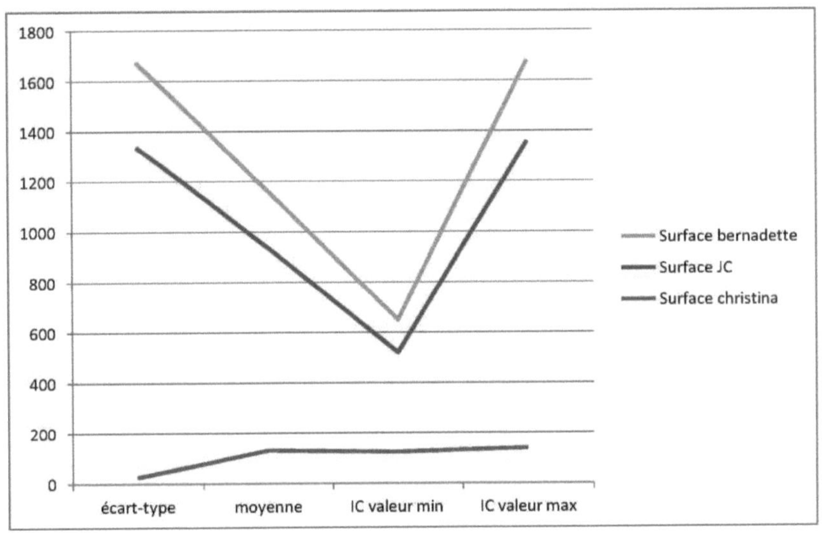

Figure22: Comparison of the surface area values of the 3 subjects

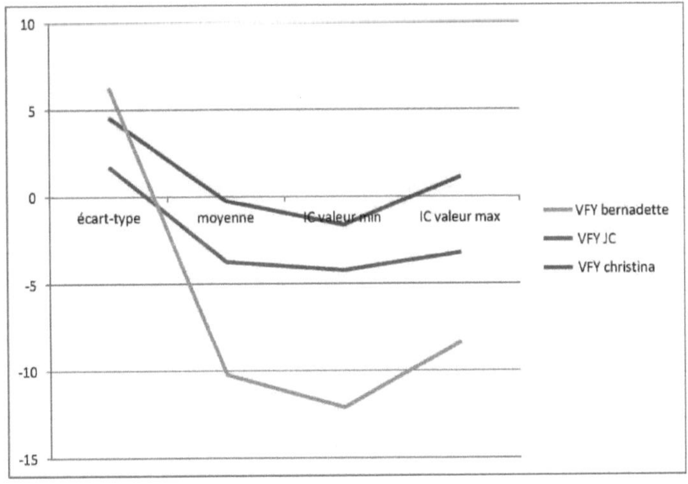

Figure 23: Comparison of the VFY values of the 3 subjects

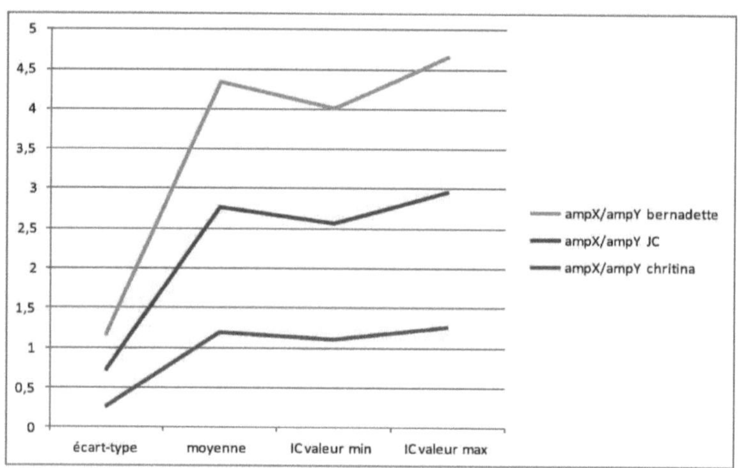

Figure 24: comparison of ampX/ampY values of the 3 subjects

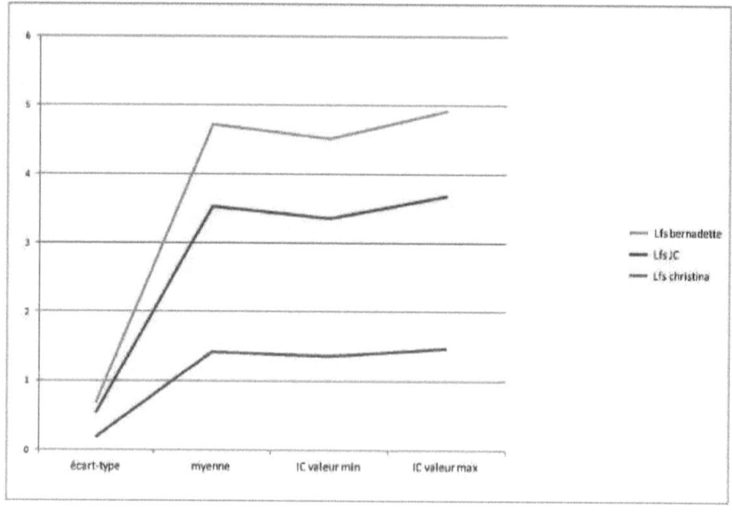

Figure 25 Comparison of the LFS values of the 3 subjects

A. Objectives of the study

From the previous results, it has been shown that each subject is independent and has its own values, so it seems impossible on subjects who complain of occluso-posturo disorders, to say whether their results are "normal" or not.

Thirty subjects were selected from Dr Combadazou's patient file, the choice was made in alphabetical order to avoid introducing selection bias. These thirty patients were referred by posturologists, osteopaths, physiotherapists because they presented postural pain and all felt an improvement after treatment with a gutter.

The main objective of this study is to see whether this subjective improvement is reflected in the recordings.

B. Material and method

1) <u>Sample</u>

Recruitment of patients was done as previously mentioned, i.e. in alphabetical order, regardless of gender, and they all had to have felt an improvement.

2) <u>The recordings</u>

The occlusal disorders were diagnosed on the basis of a clinical examination and with the help of recordings made with the Myotronics® K7 system, which allows the simultaneous recording of mandibular movements and the activity of the mandibular muscles.

The registrations with the standardised SATEL platform have been carried out

- From 2 and a half to 9 months after wearing gutters with an average of 5 3/4 months.
- If the patients have inserts, they have kept them.
- Eyes closed.
- A recording is made in the mandibular posture (resting position) and then with the teeth clenched.

Registrations <u>ANNEX 4</u>

Example of registration <u>ANNEX 5</u>

3) <u>Statistics</u>

In this study, we compare the results of a treatment for each individual in the sample. This is a qualitative study and not a quantitative one.

In the previous experiment, we found that the results were significant intra-person but not inter-person, in this experiment we will try to see if there is an improvement after wearing the gutter, without comparing the subjects with each other, just the results before and during the treatment. It is therefore a qualitative and not a quantitative result.

To do this, we will use the matched test of Wilcoxon's ranks, setting the significance threshold at 5% thanks to the site ***marne.u707.jussieu.fr/biostatgv/?module=tests.***

This test will allow us to compare two measurements of a quantitative variable carried out on the same subjects (measurements defined by the modalities of the qualitative variable).

That is to say, it will take all the data and classify them into a series of numbers with a "label" before and after each one. A significant result will be obtained if the distributions are shifted (for example more forward for high values).

It should be noted that, in our study, the effect of the gutter will be significant when p is less than 0.05.

We therefore carried out the Wilcoxon test on :

- The surface area
- The Xaverage
- The VfY
- The LFS
- AmpX/AmpY

C. Results

1) <u>**Wilcoxon test results in mandibular posture**</u>

Here the test will compare the influence of the gutter on the mandibular posture.

	Value of p
Surface	0,23665234446526
Lfs	0,73425767427034
VfY	0,48984608799219
Xmoyen	0,28942605908184
AmpX/AmpY	0,28942605908184

We can see that in mandibular posture the data are not **significant.** This result is in fact normal because there is no reason for the gutter to influence the mandibular posture as there is no dento-dental contact.

2) <u>**Wilcoxon test result tight teeth**</u>

Here the test compares the influence of the gutter on the tight teeth.

	Value of p
Surface	0,023410143330693
Lfs	0,765495215103400
Vfy	0,855271723121400
Xmoyen	0,190929520875220
AmpX/Ampy	0,071895812493212

The data here are only significant for the area with a p less than 0.05.

It is also observed that the AmpX/AmpY ratio is close to the number 0.05, with a p equal to 0.07 (to the nearest tenth).

3) **Cohen's result d**

The calculation of Cohen's d will allow us to calculate the size of the effect, i.e. to assess the effect of the orthoses on the surface, even if the surface is a significant factor.

Cohen considers that the effect is weak for a d=0.2, average for a d=0.5 and strong for a d=0.8.

group A surface before treatment	group B surface after treatment
Area A	Surface B
848,91959	451,82283
207,51844	242,12324
147,60963	68,68275
163,77629	148,7169
334,99387	830,25503
376,2858	123,9553
393,98992	241,77142
732,41976	508,77898
407,8057	304,89149
490,25942	403,21326
153,10238	316,42031
171,05939	152,5804
406,60494	371,52578
345,23526	258,31158
391,54847	414,05051
82,66877	122,38378
513,3594	405,26871
374,68112	201,71047
533,36215	420,30449
579,86388	155,32853
160,56691	170,60592
323,30388	279,64284
339,4725	605,01545
248,67871	259,0595
101,78472	96,13119
1055,208	598,15113
228,62387	261,57475
167,93115	142,54898
237,26466	143,42969
271,25031	270,70828

d of Cohen = 0.30087808

It can be seen that the effect of the orthoses on the surface of the sustentation polygon is relatively small even if it exists.

D. Discussion

1) **The population**

The first study concerns 3 asymptomatic individuals with no proven pathology since they have never consulted for postural pain or for pain or dysfunction of the manducatory apparatus. The examinations were carried out over several days and at different time slots.

The second study concerns a selected population with both postural disorders and occlusal pathology. The diagnosis of dysocclusion is made on the basis of a clinical examination and additional tests, namely electronic recording of mandibular movements and surface EMG of the mandibular muscles.

With regard to the postural problem, the diagnosis was made by a sports doctor or an osteopath, but we did not specify the type or intensity of the postural problem. The only point of exclusion is an irreversible injury such as a herniated disc.

From the first study it appears that the results of the stabilograms are not comparable between the 3 different individuals. On the other hand, they are repetitive and comparable for each of them whatever the time of day (see V.B.2).

The two studies taken together show us that whether the first study, healthy subjects, or the second study, pathological subjects, all the values of the analysed stabilograms are within the range of normal values given by Standard 85. Our results are comparable to those of the various studies already carried out at the Toulouse dental surgery faculty (Mounet, Tournaire).

We can therefore argue that the values of Standard 85 are not sufficiently precise in the postural framework and do not a priori allow us to distinguish a patient from a healthy subject. This is corroborated by the fact that we cannot compare two individuals in order to dissociate a healthy subject from a pathological subject.

The second hypothesis of our study concerns the impact of occlusal treatments on the values obtained from the stabilometry examinations before and after the occlusal treatment; knowing that the individuals in the sample experienced an improvement in their symptoms. We note that the only parameter that can be retained is the surface area of the sustentation polygon ($p < 0.05$); on the other hand the impact on these values is small and does not seem to be related to the patients' feelings.

2) **Bias of Fétu of**

In the first part of the experiment there are 3 examiners but in the second part there is only one examiner, Dr Combadazou. Indeed the study would have been more relevant if each examination had been carried out by several examiners and several times on the same patient. This would have made it possible to calculate the inter- and intra-observer variance. The type of examination is nevertheless simple and the influence does not seem to be very important as shown in the 1st study.

For this study, we based ourselves on the patients' subjective feelings, so we cannot be sure that there is a real improvement. To reduce the subjective effect, a pain scale should have been used.

And then there are all the other inputs of the postural system which can influence the posture at the time of registration, but the examinations, in order to diminish their impact, were carried out with the eyes closed. As for the others, we trusted the correspondents who sent them to us in principle able to diagnose this type of problem. We could also have differentiated between upper pains: cervical, shoulder and arm pains, and lower pains: knee, hip, lumbar, for example.

OUTLOOK AND CONCLUSION

The aim of this study was to find out whether the use of a stabilometry platform in the context of occlusal-postural treatment was of any use.

In terms of the diagnosis of postural impairment, we can conclude that this analysis is very limited if we want to compare the values with those of Standard 85. The only usefulness is to compare the tracings of the same individual with each other, for example with eyes open and eyes closed, or with regard to dental occlusion before and after treatment, but limited to the surface study.

However, while the patient's feelings seem to show an improvement, albeit subjective, the comparison of the stabilogram plots before and after treatment is significant for only one of the six values studied: the surface of the sustentation polygon. And, the impact of the treatment on this value is small.

In conclusion, we believe that this type of examination is not very reliable for making a diagnosis and that its interest in the study of posture seems to be of little importance.

It would certainly be interesting in further studies to carry out repetitive examinations on more healthy subjects by identifying age and sex to see if for one sex and/or one age group there is a difference in values that could become norms.

APPENDIX 1

Xmoyen	Surface	Vfy	Lfs	ampX/ampY
5,44847	1428,2029	6,09242	1,59969	0,82
6,9869	2372,8137	6,55982	0,71252	1,14
8,60703	1141,9359	5,21645	1,87237	0,78
1,24512	906,10377	4,82111	1,98892	0,78
9,88718	908,22743	7,2996	2,00614	1,2
-7,01299	792,23419	0,33064	2,0434	0,78
3,40391	997,84034	6,37289	1,80119	1,05
6,76485	643,93979	3,11694	2,30977	0,96
5,28569	1031,6545	4,3823	2,02436	1,23
-10,15643	579,805	2,68876	2,60812	1,06
-1,05331	772,68924	3,33808	2,13248	1,36
6,13921	670,56685	0,30027	1,9557	1,06
6,13601	856,03527	9,11922	2,39876	0,9
0,70959	776,55031	2,71897	2,18195	0,95
-1,47727	906,51877	7,49773	2,06544	0,94
-1,92588	758,24362	5,38023	2,43211	0,92
7,48601	962,32219	6,17526	2,25908	0,79
1,4624	803,80958	4,30828	2,31462	0,99
6,0853	633,35283	5,86853	2,37524	0,84
-4,49438	661,03487	3,57516	2,3897	1,28
6,34224	826,24043	-4,06054	1,86376	0,75
-4,97576	523,83659	2,59783	2,30972	1,34
8,03964	468,19153	5,2072	2,5747	1,04
4,16986	693,20943	0,70185	2,13057	1,43
-0,20583	649,58707	0,55806	2,52768	0,92
1,12521	671,49865	-0,88475	2,10861	1,18
4,70135	729,70114	1,64838	1,81222	1,29
1,60899	685,81621	4,60321	2,12792	1,01
-0,41863	848,02561	-1,59393	1,97048	0,79
-2,63731	705,40539	6,62699	2,40311	0,77
2,33641	720,82413	1,94877	2,12363	0,79
-2,07449	675,16591	1,93051	2,10134	1,66
-5,4901	728,97039	4,70478	2,12174	1,02
-0,67802	585,60533	0,26823	2,54224	1,3
-1,13446	589,19971	6,22697	2,572	1,25
0,99624	708,59338	4,21518	2,08165	0,78
6,45217	594,21415	2,90264	2,00675	1,15
4,64304	860,12828	1,17835	1,62276	1,35
9,20134	592,20986	1,43361	1,67819	1,05

Xmoyen	Surface	Vfy	Lfs	AmpX/AmpY
6,19563	92,98274	-3,82313	1,21085	0,92
2,02977	134,49346	-6,61372	1,22555	1,23
2,48122	114,05266	-5,45795	1,22441	1,16
11,75271	157,89675	-2,54509	1,54788	1,09
7,48562	152,2963	-3,73173	1,34071	1,33
2,04904	116,32481	-4,62514	1,15745	1,16
2,11662	153,13022	-1,39201	1,30358	1,51
5,90493	102,06705	-4,7499	1,03992	1,33
6,1666	99,18086	-5,55779	1,40716	1,16
11,15404	129,76731	-5,76278	1,18751	1,24
11,40635	140,54699	-5,45836	1,37677	1,13
12,22694	152,55015	-3,91986	1,37859	1,05
4,87738	115,84992	-4,68069	1,1912	1,69
1,12585	96,45398	-4,81199	1,19641	1,05
3,00971	87,63472	-4,44471	1,21387	0,82
10,18357	131,57348	-1,86487	1,57634	1,52
5,89817	96,34397	-4,32262	1,28963	1,71
5,71256	114,91252	-4,31677	1,357	0,9
12,49452	135,15353	-5,05128	1,43748	1,38
12,02512	139,02283	-2,65913	1,45619	1,02
4,11362	140,24108	-4,12415	1,52974	1,27
5,57193	100,44952	-7,02924	1,17995	1,43
9,05417	135,34573	-4,26576	1,39252	1,09
5,60875	188,06169	-3,30102	1,49868	1,02
4,75529	129,10514	-4,87866	1,2858	1,43
5,09599	117,63306	-7,09992	1,43948	1,06
12,52663	129,10281	-1,81538	1,66939	0,9
6,37103	149,27312	-0,45918	1,39453	1
10,27869	113,19016	-1,21552	1,52019	1,81
8,32011	121,26117	-3,80576	1,52382	1
8,99746	130,2583	-1,11968	1,56465	1,04
6,25137	157,29091	-1,29958	1,71796	1,22
-1,34807	167,6958	-4,23971	1,49052	0,82
8,01644	131,25012	-0,3525	1,81476	0,99
6,98512	168,01963	-4,03547	1,72685	1,69
6,67284	130,08194	-3,95205	1,56274	0,89
9,71534	125,84854	-3,05812	1,55023	1,41
7,27253	158,55774	-3,83394	1,41324	1,48
9,81762	165,60639	-0,05652	1,70814	1,27
1,71363	119,34056	-2,18822	1,32419	1,09
3,67072	110,18223	-3,34802	1,32904	0,89
0,90724	128,46256	-5,6482	1,38801	0,79
-0,49488	171,28943	-3,6471	1,47831	1,24
1,91815	186,08618	-4,25141	1,81008	0,92
5,55467	125,23326	-3,20216	1,35085	1,26

Xmoyen	Surface	Vfy	Lfs	ampX/ampY
-2,75688	191,5579	-12,23771	1,09323	1,49
6,32685	178,13741	-10,08219	1,13772	1,4
4,54412	266,05194	-9,82592	1,16286	1,14
5,5185	143,71997	-8,5834	1,16397	1,4
8,57042	403,09712	-7,13503	0,97031	1,44
0,4475	339,42818	-9,76456	1,39986	1,36
5,37647	229,93977	-7,8912	1,15242	1,57
4,89663	201,42607	-6,88928	1,25826	1,29
2,87667	170,54478	-8,67062	1,22364	1,47
2,05588	281,90889	-8,6642	1,20451	1,46
6,20325	242,75789	-11,42777	1,34007	1,35
2,94477	342,25365	-7,04455	1,11324	2,33
3,3869	181,29249	-8,97119	1,1245	0,92
-0,14043	204,11923	-9,58776	1,20173	1,64
2,286	229,2958	-10,12024	1,20329	1,23
2,77955	209,78354	-8,07677	1,20728	1,25
-0,89531	119,6549	-10,25688	0,92885	1,46
0,11026	241,22389	-11,34662	1,03768	1,71
6,56926	198,42452	-10,53398	1,14968	1,33
4,54307	201,34092	-10,27482	1,14161	1,43
-1,46876	223,75933	-10,58989	1,20676	1,72
2,95012	167,64157	-10,43054	1,1795	1,26
1,95605	144,08972	-8,16359	1,38146	2,07
-4,01206	125,2961	-11,60176	1,1299	1,42
1,52073	188,61929	-9,02586	1,18466	2,08
4,28736	238,73955	-10,83621	1,21755	1,08
4,53272	186,20751	-8,26822	1,10537	2,28
1,77878	323,02151	-10,40296	1,16359	2,71
-4,91803	134,46888	-10,85184	1,0084	2,33
0,58165	160,77999	-11,26766	1,10242	1,17
-6,06317	218,31908	-11,36866	1,08364	1,63
0,63647	229,65974	-10,7486	1,17683	1,6
2,43775	132,61389	-11,06943	1,17722	1,82
-2,73173	108,9838	-12,0141	1,16717	1,95
7,49941	148,48755	-12,11668	1,14675	1,03
-1,73788	162,7875	-10,26106	1,16584	2,11
3,9027	235,71447	-11,77542	1,20899	1,5
1,67694	200,96739	-8,05263	1,19741	2
3,55267	202,21753	-12,80937	1,21245	1,05
0,11726	144,90658	-8,30138	1,34215	1,1
1,97186	279,03225	-8,06407	1,18088	1,66
8,52839	790,23057	-6,171	1,02468	2,94
1,50979	248,28072	-14,05774	1,39418	1,56
3,60482	281,48562	-12,55227	1,67696	1,15
2,31064	185,17903	-10,34031	1,29955	1,46
2,15307	326,82364	-10,45449	1,62179	1,15

APPENDIX 4

Patient Name	Sex	Heure Enreg	Frequence Enreg	Situa Vis Enreg	Situa Pod Enreg	Situa Mand Enreg	Duree Enreg	Taille Enreg	Pointure Enreg	Surface	Xmoyen	Ymoyen	Lfs	Vfy	AmpX/AmpY
Patient 1	Male	15:58:14	40	YF	Sole	sture mandibulai	51,2	1,78	43	367	-8,4562	-23,143	2	7,5	2,72
	Male	15:59:34	40	YF	Sole	i serrées engrén.	51,2	1,78	43	848,92	-8,7936	-14,558	1	7,5	1,23
	Male	12:31:48	40	YF	Sole	e mandib with gold	51,2	1,78	43	319,5	1,09394	-14,792	2	3,2	2,18
	Male	12:33:08	40	YF	Sole	serrées max. ort	51,2	1,78	43	451,82	-1,2271	-11,557	1	2,4	1,49
Patient 2	Female	10:00:55	40	YF	Sole	sture mandibulai	51,2	1,66	39	313,45	8,40924	-22,394	1	1,5	2,14
	Female	10:02:29	40	YF	Sole	i serrées engrén.	51,2	1,66	39	207,52	9,34779	-24,911	1	-2	0,96
	Female	16:47:37	40	YF	Sole	e mandib with gold	51,2	1,66	39	246,62	2,0294	-14,267	1	0,5	1,17
	Female	16:49:00	40	YF	Sole	serrées max. ort	51,2	1,66	39	242,12	8,84668	-15,422	1	-0	1,67
Patient 3	Female	10:34:46	40	YF	On hard ground	sture mandibulai	51,2	1,77	39	169,05	9,47235	-28,356	1	-5	1,27
	Female	10:35:51	40	YF	On hard ground	; serrated engendered.	51,2	1,77	39	147,61	7,96906	-26,439	1	-6	0,81
	Female	10:13:21	40	YF	On hard ground	e mandib with gold	51,2	1,77	39	126	4,77559	-36,649	1	-7	2,99
	Female	10:28:33	40	YF	On hard ground	serrées max. ort	51,2	1,77	39	68,683	6,58466	-25,728	1	-5	1,18
Patient 4	Female	11:45:47	40	YF	Sole	sture mandibulai	51,2	1,65	39	140,71	0,14848	-22,892	1	-3	1,04
	Female	11:46:59	40	YF	Sole	i serrées engrén.	51,2	1,65	39	163,78	3,55624	-28,623	1	-5	2,23
	Female	14:11:30	40	YF	Sole	e mandib w th gold	51,2	1,65	39	204,73	9,82374	-26,489	1	-3	1,06
	Female	14:12:48	40	YF	Sole	serrées max. ort	51,2	1,65	39	148,72	13,5298	-22,878	1	-4	1,18
Patient 5	Male	11:29:07	40	YF	On hard ground	sture mandibulai	51,2	1,84	44	447,47	-9,5272	-51,585	1	-8	2,07
	Male	11:30:13	40	YF	On hard ground	i serrées engrén.	51,2	1,84	44	334,99	-6,1917	-34,679	1	-4	0,96
	Male	12:12:59	40	YF	On hard ground	s tightened max. m	51,2	1,84	44	635,54	9,71761	-21,141	1	-1	1,02
	Male	12:46:47	40	YF	On hard ground	serrées max. ort	51,2	1,84	44	830,26	5,02717	-37,453	1	-2	1,3
	Male	12:48:57	40	YF	On hard ground	e mandib with gold	51,2	1,84	44	1184,2	4,58703	-37,615	1	-3	1,9
Patient 6	Female	15:46:32	40	YF	On hard ground	sture mandibulai	51,2	1,74	40	465,36	5,68361	-38,674	1	-6	0,85
	Female	15:48:04	40	YF	On hard ground	; serrated engendered.	51,2	1,74	40	376,29	-9,5919	-34,305	1	-5	0,69
	Female	09:26:21	40	YF	On hard ground	e mandib with gold	51,2	1,74	40	245,55	-2,2645	-46,429	1	-7	1,13
	Female	09:27:44	40	YF	On hard ground	serrées max. ort	51,2	1,74	40	217,38	-5,3143	-37,507	1	-4	1,21

| | Female | 09:13:49 | 40 | YF | On hard ground | e mandib with gold | 51,2 | 1,74 | 40 | 294,92 | -1,0414 | -41,435 | 1 | -6 | 0,87 |
| | Female | 09:15:04 | 40 | YF | On hard ground | serrées max. ort | 51,2 | 1,74 | 40 | 123,96 | -2,2464 | -34,995 | 1 | -5 | 1,24 |

Patient 7	Male	10:41:43	40	YF	On hard ground	sture mandibulai	51,2	1,82	43	284,53	-1,2241	-45,208	2	-4	1,24
	Male	10:43:43	40	YF	On hard ground	s tightened max. m	51,2	1,82	43	393,99	-3,0483	-41,967	2	-3	1,4
	Male	09:06:56	40	YF	On hard ground	e mandib with gold	51,2	1,82	43	505,86	-2,7518	-55,638	1	-10	1,3
	Male	09:08:29	40	YF	On hard ground	serrées max. ort	51,2	1,82	43	241,77	-3,8576	-56,481	1	-12	0,98
Patient 8	Female	14:28:19	40	YF	On hard ground	sture mandibulai	51,2	1,65	37	713,93	6,30341	-55,078	1	-7	1,62
	Female	14:29:37	40	YF	On hard ground	i serrées engrén.	51,2	1,65	37	732,42	4,91256	-50,989	1	-6	0,8
	Female	14:10:41	40	YF	On hard ground	e mandib with gold	51,2	1,65	37	474,58	13,6333	-43,268	1	-5	1,08
	Female	14:12:32	40	YF	On hard ground	serrées max. ort	51,2	1,65	37	508,78	11,004	-49,454	1	-7	1,39
Patient 9	Female	09:17:58	40	YF	On hard ground	sture mandibulai	51,2	1,67	37	527,9	0,41902	-50,519	1	-7	1,09
	Female	09:19:14	40	YF	On hard ground	i serrées engrén.	51,2	1,67	37	407,81	-0,471	-48,552	1	-6	0,97
	Female	15:43:34	40	YF	On hard ground	e mandib with gold	51,2	1,67	37	714,98	2,97877	-59,725	1	-11	1,03
	Female	15:44:52	40	YF	On hard ground	serrées max. ort	51,2	1,67	37	304,89	3,19049	-42,218	1	-6	0,78
Patient 10	Female	12:15:11	40	YF	On hard ground	sture mandibulai	51,2	1,63	40	600,73	-3,2879	-58,249	1	-7	1,54
	Female	12:16:26	40	YF	On hard ground	i serrées engrén.	51,2	1,63	40	490,26	-2,3441	-59,037	2	-7	1,01
	Female	12:00:15	40	YF	Sole	e mandib with gold	51,2	1,63	40	561,63	2,82021	-19,288	1	3,4	3
	Female	12:01:52	40	YF	Sole	serrées max. ort	51,2	1,63	40	403,21	0,07782	-15,041	1	2,3	1,96
Patient 11	Female	14:23:06	40	YF	Sole	sture mandibulai	51,2	1,57	37	142,77	-3,0498	-39,522	1	-7	1,37
	Female	14:24:27	40	YF	Sole	serrated	51,2	1,57	37	153,1	-5,9721	-35,508	1	-6	1,34
	Female	15:49:35	40	YF	Sole	e mandib with gold	51,2	1,57	37	215,54	2,54911	-56,754	1	-10	2,25
	Female	15:50:55	40	YF	Sole	serrées max. ort	51,2	1,57	37	316,42	0,79645	-58,164	1	-10	2,25
Patient 12	Female	17:09:03	40	YF	On hard ground	sture mandibulai	51,2	1,65	37	268,83	8,80896	-50,839	2	-0	2,08
	Female	17:10:18	40	YF	On hard ground	i serrées engrén.	51,2	1,65	37	171,06	9,59959	-53,197	2	-8	1,41
	Female	12:00:46	40	YF	On hard ground	e mandib with gold	51,2	1,65	37	228,24	2,75439	-48,626	1	-9	1,31
	Female	12:02:11	40	YF	On hard ground	serrées max. ort	51,2	1,65	37	178,65	7,53733	-44,885	1	-8	1,03
	Female	12:04:45	40	YF	Sole	e mandib with gold	51,2	1,65	37	203,64	6,16542	-30,802	1	-1	1,4
	Female	12:06:03	40	YF	Sole	serrées max. ort	51,2	1,65	37	152,58	9,07535	-35,431	1	-3	1,08

Patient 13	Male	16:34:04	40	YF	Sole	sture mandibulai	51,2	1,7	41	524,11	-10,802	-28,3	1	0,2	1,62
	Male	16:35:21	40	YF	Sole	i serrées engrén.	51,2	1,7	41	406,6	-8,6144	-21,779	1	0,4	0,93
	Male	14:08:12	40	YF	Sole	e mandib with gold	51,2	1,7	41	253,83	-1,9274	-26,928	2	-1	1,79
	Male	14:09:32	40	YF	Sole	serrées max. ort	51,2	1,7	41	371,53	-2,8617	-14,861	1	0,7	3,16
Patient 14	Male	17:01:13	40	YF	On hard ground	sture mandibulai	51,2	1,78	43	218,32	4,71555	-23,258	2	-1	1,65
	Male	17:02:34	40	YF	Sole	; serrated	51,2	1,78	43	345,24	4,41916	-15,487	1	0,1	1,07
	Male	12:25:45	40	YF	Sole	e mandib with gold	51,2	1,78	43	214,21	1,68101	-22,309	2	0,5	1,53
	Male	12:27:12	40	YF	Sole	serrées max. ort	51,2	1,78	43	178,74	9,24794	-27,618	2	-2	1,11
	Male	12:32:23	40	YF	Sole	e mandib with gold	51,2	1,78	43	211,18	5,17323	-30,967	1	-2	1,03
	Male	12:33:37	40	YF	Sole	serrées max. ort	51,2	1,78	43	258,31	12,1395	-28,707	2	-2	1,35
Patient 15	Female	15:48:17	40	YF	On hard ground	sture mandibulai	51,2	1,62	38	384,49	0,27189	-26,517	1	-1	1,21
	Female	15:49:39	40	YF	On hard ground	i serrées engrén.	51,2	1,62	38	391,55	-1,4307	-27,174	1	-4	0,9
	Female	10:34:57	40	YF	On hard ground	e mandib with gold	51,2	1,62	38	318,63	0,70562	-28,974	1	-3	1,18
	Female	10:36:18	40	YF	On hard ground	serrées max. ort	51,2	1,62	38	414,05	-3,8809	-33,287	1	-4	1,13
Patient 16	Female	16:57:08	40	YF	On hard ground	sture mandibulai	51,2	1,62	38	150,71	-5,9639	-39,687	1	-6	1,23
	Female	16:58:29	40	YF	On hard ground	i serrées engrén.	51,2	1,62	38	82,669	-10,184	-42,512	1	-9	1,06
	Female	18:48:49	40	YF	On hard ground	e mandib with gold	51,2	1,62	38	219,86	2,2938	-39,012	1	-8	1,4
	Female	18:50:04	40	YF	On hard ground	serrées max. ort	51,2	1,62	38	122,38	-0,0353	-40,541	1	-9	1
Patient 17	Female	18:24:24	40	YF	On hard ground	sture mandibulai	51,2	1,68	38	1178,6	4,31731	-52,894	1	-4	1,04
	Female	18:26:00	40	YF	On hard ground	i serrées engrén.	51,2	1,68	38	513,36	-0,1465	-52,798	1	-8	1,24
	Female	18:13:48	40	YF	On hard ground	e mandib with gold	51,2	1,68	38	796,31	-7,5205	-51,329	1	-3	1,71
	Female	18:15:19	40	YF	On hard ground	serrées max. ort	51,2	1,68	38	405,27	-6,3266	-44,886	2	-3	1,12
Patient 18	Male	16:32:03	40	YF	Sole	sture mandibulai	51,2	1,75	44	300,07	5,70287	-28,257	1	-2	1,58
	Male	16:33:23	40	YF	Sole	; serrated	51,2	1,75	44	374,68	8,24599	-23,993	1	-1	1,3
	Male	12:21:59	40	YF	On hard ground	e mandib with gold	51,2	1,75	44	448,36	0,27383	-33,487	2	9,9	0,64
	Male	12:23:22	40	YF	On hard ground	serrées max. ort	51,2	1,75	44	327,33	-0,1591	-31,112	1	-1	1,13
	Male	15:48:28	40	YO	On hard ground	e mandib with gold	51,2	1,75	44	213,33	-7,0703	-46,772	2	-3	1,16
	Male	15:50:08	40	YO	On hard ground	serrées max. ort	51,2	1,75	44	75,238	1,94969	-46,76	1	-11	0,71

Male	15:51:40	40	YF	On hard ground	e mandib with gold	51,2	1,75	44	277,06	-0,3891	-47,171	1	-9	1,9
Male	15:52:49	40	YF	On hard ground	serrées max. ort	51,2	1,75	44	201,71	-2,7415	-50,964	1	-11	1,48

Patient 19	Male	16:58:45	40	YF	On hard ground	sture mandibulai	51,2	1,85	43	681,14	6,58137	-44,365	1	-3	1,42
	Male	17:00:05	40	YF	On hard ground	i serrées engrén.	51,2	1,85	43	533,36	1,81226	-51,322	2	-6	1,52
	Male	16:57:00	40	YF	On hard ground	e mandib with gold	51,2	1,85	43	445,11	-0,6416	-47,649	2	-5	1,3
	Male	16:58:20	40	YF	On hard ground	serrées max. ort	51,2	1,85	43	420,3	0,60584	-48,199	2	-6	1,26
Patient 20	Male	17:00:29	40	YF	Sole	sture mandibulai	51,2	1,9	46	476,67	7,3329	-45,061	1	-3	2,14
	Male	17:01:49	40	YF	Sole	i serrées engrén.	51,2	1,9	46	579,86	1,13056	-43,222	1	-6	1,99
	Male	17:40:29	40	YF	On hard ground	e mandib with gold	51,2	1,9	46	353,76	2,17168	-60,538	1	-10	0,91
	Male	17:41:49	40	YF	On hard ground	serrées max. ort	51,2	1,9	46	155,33	0,757	-53,48	1	-9	0,97
Patient 21	Female	16:25:21	40	YF	On hard ground	sture mandibulai	51,2	1,75	40	188,05	-3,4832	-47,217	1	-10	2,06
	Female	16:26:47	40	YF	On hard ground	i serrées engrén.	51,2	1,75	40	160,57	-1,1279	-49,036	1	-10	1,38
	Female	18:42:57	40	YF	On hard ground	e mandib with gold	51,2	1,75	40	151,42	-1,8411	-44,628	1	-7	1,61
	Female	18:44:21	40	YF	On hard ground	serrées max. ort	51,2	1,75	40	170,61	-1,251	-42,267	1	-8	1,23
Patient 22	Male	14:28:21	40	YF	On hard ground	sture mandibulai	51,2	1,73	42	226,86	5,79133	-59,81	1	-14	1,56
	Male	14:29:37	40	YF	On hard ground	; serrated	51,2	1,73	42	323,3	7,09517	-51,631	1	-11	0,97
	Male	17:04:36	40	YF	Sole	e mandib with gold	51,2	1,73	42	132,51	8,04116	-32,916	1	-6	1,19
	Male	17:06:08	40	YF	Sole	serrées max. ort	51,2	1,73	42	279,64	7,72297	-37,265	1	-8	0,95
Patient 23	Male	16:33:24	40	YF	On hard ground	sture mandibulai	51,2	1,6	37	330,54	3,90388	-25,247	2	1,5	0,95
	Male	16:34:33	40	YF	On hard ground	i serrées engrén.	51,2	1,75	43	339,47	5,04413	-38,238	2	-3	0,81
	Male	09:34:12	40	YF	On hard ground	e mandib with gold	51,2	1,75	43	882,46	1,45724	-59,918	1	-5	2,28
	Male	09:35:41	40	YF	On hard ground	serrées max. ort	51,2	1,75	43	605,02	1,98261	-56,398	1	-8	1,12
Patient 24	Male	18:05:35	40	YF	On hard ground	sture mandibulai	51,2	1,78	43	275,69	1,67145	-51,907	1	-10	1,13
	Male	18:06:52	40	YF	On hard ground	; serrated	51,2	1,78	43	248,68	2,97018	-56,241	1	-11	1,05
	Male	09:18:56	40	YF	On hard ground	e mandib with gold	51,2	1,78	43	527,69	2,41417	-38,765	1	-5	1,05
	Male	09:20:10	40	YF	On hard ground	serrées max. ort	51,2	1,78	43	259,06	1,42339	-45,577	1	-8	2,07

Patient 25	Female	14:52:46	40	YF	On hard ground	sture mandibulai	51,2	1,6	38	187,64	0,82856	-39,186	2	-5	1,46
	Female	14:54:17	40	YF	On hard ground	i serrées engrén.	51,2	1,6	38	101,78	1,41753	-29,993	1	-4	1,39
	Female	14:27:57	40	YF	Sole	e mandib with gold	51,2	1,6	38	210,87	-2,9933	-12,489	1	-1	1,31
	Female	14:29:22	40	YF	Sole	serrées max. ort	51,2	1,6	38	96,131	-8,3454	-6,667	1	-1	1,5
Patient 26	Female	12:14:20	40	YF	On hard ground	sture mandibulai	51,2	1,69	39	363,41	-0,8813	-10,468	1	-1	0,66
	Female	12:15:40	40	YF	On hard ground	i serrées engrén.	51,2	1,69	39	1055,2	33,9774	-26,798	1	-3	0,73
	Female	12:56:51	40	YF	On hard ground	e mandib with gold	51,2	1,69	39	269,66	-2,0872	-15,628	1	-1	1,02
	Female	12:58:06	40	YF	On hard ground	serrées max. ort	51,2	1,69	39	598,15	1,9466	3,11739	1	1,1	1,94
Patient 27	Male	17:18:33	40	YF	Sole	sture mandibulai	51,2	1,82	45	491,49	-8,1059	-41,462	1	-6	1,51
	Male	17:20:02	40	YF	Sole	i serrées engrén.	51,2	1,82	45	228,62	-0,4714	-28,096	1	-3	1,55
	Male	18:28:50	40	YF	Sole	e mandib with gold	51,2	1,82	45	319,13	3,54264	-41,694	1	-7	0,98
	Male	18:30:15	40	YF	Sole	serrées max. ort	51,2	1,82	45	261,57	4,61194	-35,517	1	-5	1,08
Patient 28	Female	09:21:26	40	YF	On hard ground	sture mandibulai	51,2	1,72	39	359,99	-9,6116	-10,066	1	1,5	2,57
	Female	09:22:41	40	YF	On hard ground	; serrated engendered.	51,2	1,72	39	167,93	-16,365	-8,3783	1	-1	1,43
	Female	18:48:20	40	YF	On hard ground	e mandib with gold	51,2	1,72	39	207,04	-1,0771	-31,761	2	-1	1,25
	Female	18:50:05	40	YF	On hard ground	serrées max. ort	51,2	1,72	39	142,55	-7,9656	-26,296	1	-3	1,52
Patient 29	Male	11:57:52	40	YF	On hard ground	sture mandibulai	51,2	1,75	42	146,76	4,24945	-60,386	1	-12	2,04
	Male	11:59:09	40	YF	On hard ground	i serrées engrén.	51,2	1,75	42	237,26	1,23079	-47,367	1	-8	1,51
	Male	12:07:58	40	YF	On hard ground	e mandib with gold	51,2	1,75	42	108,41	7,49209	-44,736	1	-9	1,17
	Male	12:09:12	40	YF	On hard ground	serrées max. ort	51,2	1,75	42	136,35	2,63075	-41,845	1	-9	2,38
	Male	12:48:00	40	YF	On hard ground	e mandib with gold	51,2	1,75	42	159,44	5,95095	-48,997	1	-10	1,39
	Male	12:49:07	40	YF	On hard ground	serrées max. ort	51,2	1,75	42	143,43	1,91514	-40,47	1	-8	1,5
Patient 30	Male	12:25:39	40	YF	On hard ground	sture mandibu ai	51,2	1,9	44	407	3,78701	-37,16	1	-4	1,78
	Male	12:26:52	40	YF	On hard ground	i serrées engrén.	51,2	1,9	44	271,25	2,61476	-30,031	1	-4	1,18
	Male	12:46:50	40	YF	On hard ground	e mandib with gold	51,2	1,9	44	338,07	12,0393	-24,932	1	-2	0,97
	Male	12:48:00	40	YF	On hard ground	serrées max. ort	51,2	1,9	44	270,71	16,9576	-29,862	1	-4	1,68

73

Evaluation of equilibrium in static condition YF

Satel

Patient : DJOAR Melanie
Date of birth 01/05/1996
W Social Security :
Pathology: Healthy subject

Prescriber . COMBADAZOU Jean Claude
Occlusodontiste
34, rue de Metz
31000 TOULOUSE Tél: 05-61-52-63-69

Examination *W* 1051 of 19/04/2012 at 12.15pm

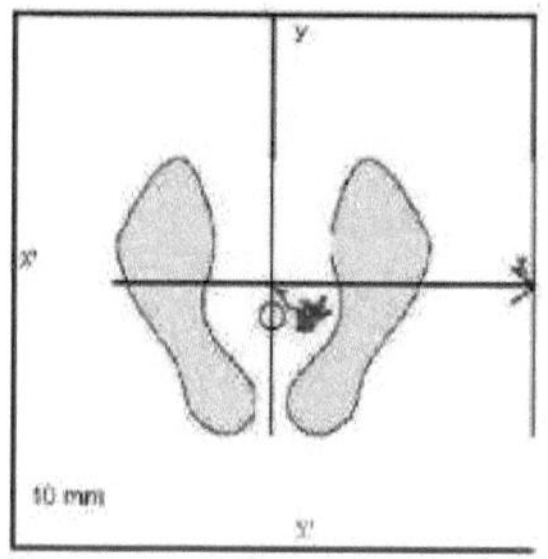

X Moyen Y	: 33,98 mm	0,3(-10,5/ 11,1)
Moyen	: -26,80 mm	-27,5 (-3,6 / -51,4)
Longueur	: 564,94 mm	613 (346 / 880)
Surface	: 1055,21 mm²	225 (79 / 638)
Longueur X	: 390,81 mm	317 (194 / 440)
Amp X	: 55,02 mm	(18 / 29)
Longueur Y	: 327,93 mm	480 (280 / 680)
Amp Y	: 40,04 mm	(27 / 45)
Ly/Lx	: 0,84	(1,3 / 1,5)
LFS adulte	: 0,52	1 (0,70 / 1,44)
Prédo. directionnelle	: 146,43	Trige.
VFY	: -4,92	
Coef. de Romberg	: NC	288 (112 /677)

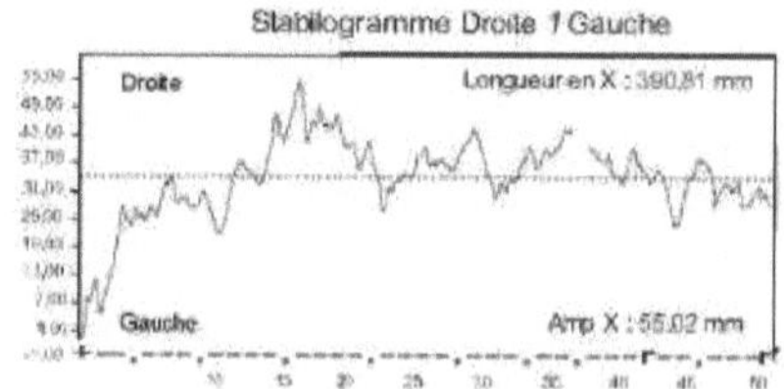

Stabilogramme Droite / Gauche

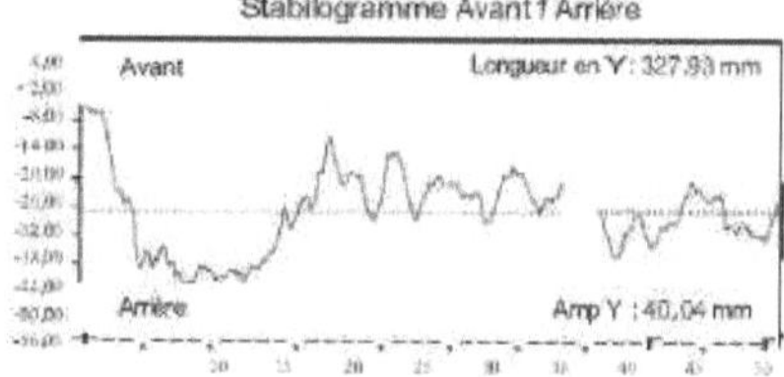

Stabilogramme Avant / Arrière

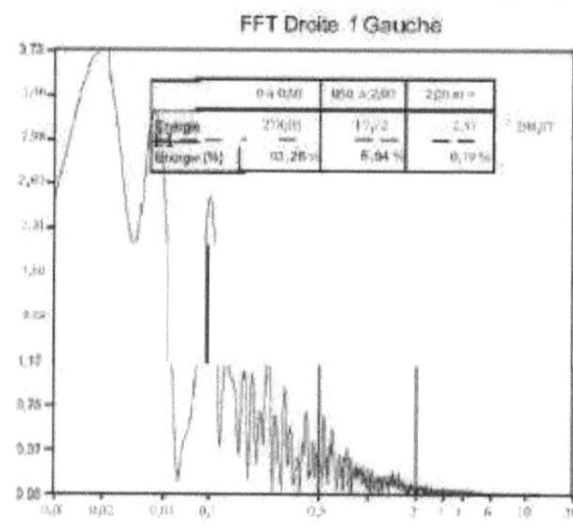

FFT Droite / Gauche

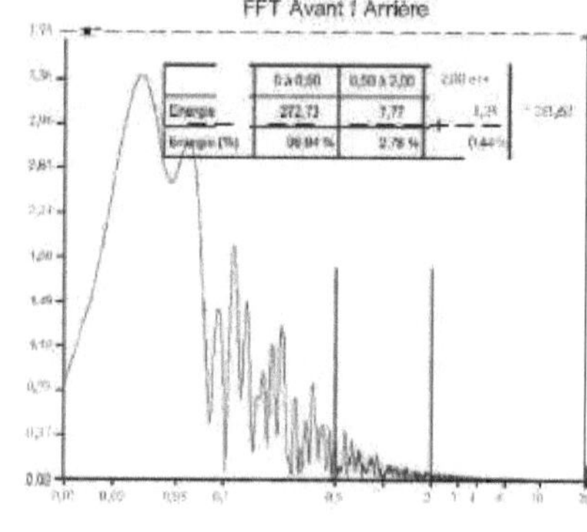

FFT Avant / Arrière

Conditions d'examen

Fréquence: 40,0 Hz
Durée : 51,2 s
Plantaire : Sur sol dur

Vestibulaire : Sans
Occlusale : Dents serrées engrén. max.
Rachidienne : Sans
Autre : Sans

Critère 1 .
Critère 2:
Critère 3 -

Thesis of Doctor Louis MOUNET

The inclusion criteria for the study were :
- L2 and D1 students from the Faculty of Dental Surgery in Toulouse,
- The age of the subjects studied was between 20 and 25 years old,

The criteria for non-inclusion were :
- the subject should not have undergone any orthodontic treatment, i.e. present a naturally healthy occlusion from any intervention.
- the subject's facial hair must not interfere with the surface electromyographic recordings.

No gender distinction was made

	Tight teeth					
	Surface		X average		Ymoyen	
	Healthy	Patho.	Healthy	Patho.	Healthy	Patho.
Average	191,7578947	247,91875	-0,86947368	0,7925	-44,68842105	-41,641875
Deviation Type	86,72549347	142,3303802	6,320028546	6,850200484	13,26166583	16,4146496
Mann-Whitney	0.3011		0.4032		0.7069	

Table: Results of comparison of stabilometric analysis of healthy and pathological subjects during closed-eye exercise with the mandible relaxed.

INFORMED CONSENT

I, the undersigned, ... declare that I   have been informed by Miss ROUMIGUIE

nasturtium, student in dental surgery and by Dr JC COMBADAZOU, of all the data concerning this research.

I accept that my recordings on the stabilometry table made at Dr COMBADAZOU's are used.

I declare that I am signing this consent, of my own free will, without any pressure, and in full possession of my means.

Last name, First name ....

BIBLIOGRAPHY

1. the myostabilised centred relationship. March 2008;(141). Available at: http://www.sop.asso.fr/admin/documents/supportfic/FDC0000019/Conseils_pratiques_en_Oc c lusodontie_-_SOP.pdf

2. Orthlieb J-D. Practical occlusodontics. Wolters Kluwer France; 2000. 240 p.

3. Tounemouly C. Occlusion and posture: neuro-anatomo-physiological links and postural pathologies [Exercise thesis]. France]: Paul Sabatier University (Toulouse). Faculty of dental surgery; 2009.

4. B. Tavernier, J. Romerowski, E. Boccara, C. Azevedo, G. Bresson. Tooth articulation and occlusal function.

5. A. Rub and B. Tavernier. synthesis:Occlusal functions: physiological aspects of human dental occlusion.

6. Josépha BALLAND. Management of the vertical dimension in the bruxomane.

7. Introduction to Therapeutic Occlusion ~ [Dental Scientific Club] [Internet]. cited 12 Oct 2015] [cited 12 Oct 2015]. Available at: http://csd23.blogspot.fr/2009/04/introduction-locclusion- therapeutique.html

8. Gaspard M. Dental occlusion disorders and S.A.D.A.M.: commented semiology and discussed etiopathogeny of the algo-dysfunctional syndrome of the manducatory apparatus: therapeutic orientations. Procodif; 1985. 280 p.

9. Orthlieb J-D, Brocard D, Schittly J, Manière-Ezvan A. Practical occlusodontics. Ruel-Malmaison France: Editions CdP; 2006. 213 p.

10. Franco AL, de Andrade MF, Segalla JCM, de Godoi Gonçalves DA, Camparis CM. New Approaches to Dental Occlusion: A Literature Update. CRANIO J Craniomandib Sleep Pract. Apr 2012;30(2):136-43.

11. Gibbs CH, Mahan PE, Lundeen HC, Brehnan K, Walsh EK, Holbrook WB. Occlusal forces during chewing and swallowing as measured by sound transmission. J Prosthet Dent. oct 1981;46(4):443-9.

12. Valentin CM, Morin F. [Maximal intercuspation: clinical examination. Characteristics of maximal intercuspation]. Cah Prothèse. avr 1982;10(38):101 -16.

13. Clauzade M, Marty J-P. Orthoposturodontics 2. Seoo Editions; 2007. 218 p.

14. Gagey P-M, Weber B. Posturology: regulation and disturbance of the standing position. Elsevier Masson; 2005. 230 p.

15. Busquet L. Les chaînes musculaires: Tome 1, Trunk, cervical spine and upper limbs, 5th edition. Frison-Roche; 2000. 159 p.

16. Robert P, Rey A, Rey-Debove J. Le Nouveau Petit Robert: alphabetical and analogical dictionary of the French language. Dictionaries Le Robert; 2012. book p.

17. faculty of medicine pierre and marie curie. FMPMC-PS - Functional Anatomy - Psychomotricity second year [Internet]. cited 21 Apr 2015]. Available at: http://www.chups.jussieu.fr/polysPSM/anatfonctPSM2/poly/POLY.Chp.3.html

18. Blayac JP. Posture, balance and rehabilitation medicine. Masson; 1993. 308 p.

19. Bricot B. Global postural reprogramming. Sauramps medical; 2009. 248 p.

20. Kamina P. Anatomy Notebook Volume 2 - Head, neck, back. MALOINE; 2014. 129 p.

21. Busquet L. Muscle chains: Volume 2, Lordoses, Cyphosis, Scoliosis and Thoracic deformations. Editions Frison-Roche; 1998. 198 p.

22. Schwegler J, Lucius R. The Human Body: Anatomical and Physiological Basis. Maloine; 2013. 450 p.

23. J. CASALI. Muscle chains according to L.busquet. 2004.

24. Perinetti G. Dental occlusion and body posture: No detectable correlation. Gait Posture. oct 2006;24(2):165-8.

25. Manfredini D, Castroflorio T, Perinetti G, Guarda-Nardini L. Dental occlusion, body posture and temporomandibular disorders: where we are now and where we are heading for. J Oral Rehabil. juin 2012;39(6):463 - 71.

26. van't Spijker A, Creugers NHJ, Bronkhorst EM, Kreulen CM. Body position and occlusal contacts in lateral excursions: a pilot study. Int J Prosthodont. avr 2011;24(2): 133-6.

27. Wakano S, Takeda T, Nakajima K, Kurokawa K, Ishigami K. Effect of experimental horizontal mandibular deviation on dynamic balance. J Prosthodont Res. oct 2011;55(4):228-33.

28. Solow B, Sonnesen L. Head posture and malocclusions. Eur J Orthod. déc 1998;20(6):685 - 93.

29. Doual JM, Ferri J, Laude M. The influence of senescence on craniofacial and cervical morphology in humans. Surg Radiol Anat SRA. 1997;19(3):175 - 83.

30. Perinetti G. Temporomandibular disorders do not correlate with detectable alterations in body posture. J Contemp Dent Pract. 2007;8(5):60-7.

31. Perinetti G, Contardo L. Posturography as a diagnostic aid in dentistry: a systematic review. J Oral Rehabil. déc 2009;36(12):922 - 36.

32. Baldini A. Clinical and instrumental treatment of a patient with dysfunction of the stomatognathic system: a case report. Ann Stomatol (Roma). avr 2010;1(2):2 -5.

33. Ohlendorf D, Seebach K, Hoerzer S, Nigg S, Kopp S. The effects of a temporarily manipulated dental occlusion on the position of the spine: a comparison during standing and

walking. Spine J. oct 2014;14(10):2384-91.

34. Miles TS, Flavel SC, Nordstrom MA. Control of human mandibular posture during locomotion. J Physiol. 1 janv 2004;554(Pt 1):216-26.

35. Dupas P-H. New approach to cranio-mandibular dysfunction: from diagnosis to the gutter. Wolters Kluwer France; 2005. 220 p.

36. Bracco P, Deregibus A, Piscetta R. Effects of different jaw relations on postural stability in human subjects. Neurosci Lett. févr 2004;356(3):228 - 30.

37. Jankelson B. Measurement accuracy of the mandibular kinesiograph--a computerized study. J Prosthet Dent. déc 1980;44(6):656 - 66.

38. Jankelson B, Swain CW, Crane PF, Radke JC. Kinesiometric instrumentation: a new technology. J Am Dent Assoc 1939. avr 1975;90(4):834 - 40.

39. Rumerio A. Tens exposure time in neuro-muscular occlusodontology: preliminary clinical study [Internet] [exercise]. Université Toulouse III - Paul Sabatier; 2014 [cited 28 Apr 2015]. Available at: http://thesesante.ups-tlse.fr/488/

40. Alwarawreh AM, Sarayreh SA, Rabadi HF, Shtaiwi Albdour EA, Al-Marzouq M. Effect of Body Posture on Malocclusion. Pak Oral Dent J. Dec 2014;34(4):635 - 9.

41. myotronics website [Internet]. Available at: http://www.myotronics.com/products/k7-evaluation- system/index.html

42. médicalxpo website [Internet]. Disponible sur: http://www.medicalexpo.fr/tab/le-systeme-k7.html?suggest=6d4c5273644447734b6544556550686465464d6a57797842354e3969507a6 b 6f68793567344c4d5761496b3d

43. site smiledentalcenterinc [Internet]. Available at: http://www.smiledentalcenterinc.com/our_technology/Kinesiograph_7_K7_evaluation_syste m. htm

44. emg [Internet]. Available at: http://www.mescan.com/systemes-d-analyse-de-l-atm/electromyography-bioemg-iii

45. Measurement in Posturology [Internet]. cited 18 May 2015]. Available at: http://ada-posturologie.fr/MesureEnPosturologie.htm

46. stat_IUT.pdf [Internet]. cited 5 Sept 2015]. Available at: https://perso.univ-rennes1.fr/jean-christophe.breton/Fichiers/stat_IUT.pdf

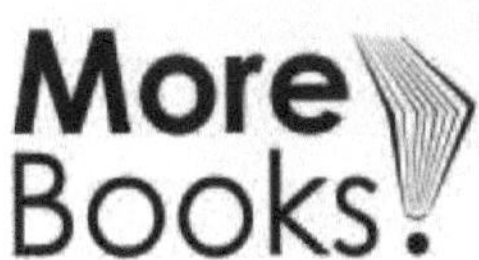

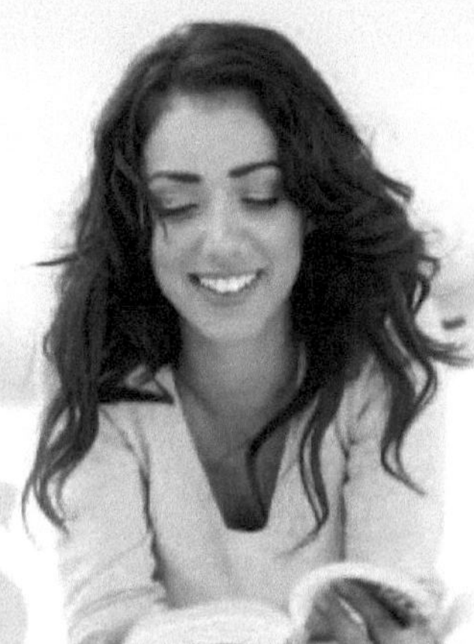

I want morebooks!

Buy your books fast and straightforward online - at one of world's fastest growing online book stores! Environmentally sound due to Print-on-Demand technologies.

Buy your books online at
www.morebooks.shop

Kaufen Sie Ihre Bücher schnell und unkompliziert online – auf einer der am schnellsten wachsenden Buchhandelsplattformen weltweit! Dank Print-On-Demand umwelt- und ressourcenschonend produzi ert.

Bücher schneller online kaufen
www.morebooks.shop

KS OmniScriptum Publishing
Brivibas gatve 197
LV-1039 Riga, Latvia
Telefax: +371 686 204 55

info@omniscriptum.com
www.omniscriptum.com

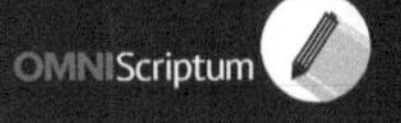

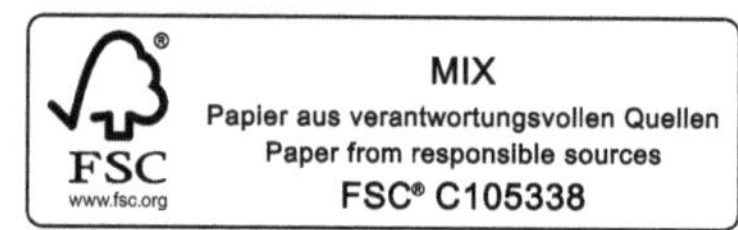